Affiliated with Molecular Biology of Hemat

AF888003

# Acta Hæmatologica

Founded 1948 by E. Meulengracht, K. Rohr, and G. Rosenow
Continued by H. Lüdin (1960–1977), U. Bucher (1977–1983), R.S. Hillman (1978–1987), H.R. Marti (1983–1988), E.A. Beck (1984–1988), B. Ramot (1989–1995)



KARGER

Printed in Switzerland on acid-free paper by Reinhardt Druck, Basel

Appears 6-weekly: 2 volumes per year (8 issues)

# Guidelines for Authors

Acta Hæmatologica

## Submission

Only original papers written in English are considered and should be sent to:

Prof. I. Ben-Bassat
S. Karger AG
Editorial Office Acta Haematologica
P.O. Box
CH–4009 Basel (Switzerland)
Tel. +41 61 306 1356
Fax +41 61 306 1434
E-Mail l.ehrsam@karger.ch

Mailing address for courier deliveries only:
Allschwilerstr. 10
CH–4055 Basel (Switzerland)

Manuscripts should be submitted in triplicate (with three sets of illustrations of which one is an original), typewritten double-spaced on one side of the paper, with a wide margin.

## Conditions

All manuscripts are subject to editorial review. Manuscripts are received with the explicit understanding that they are not under simultaneous consideration by any other publication. Submission of an article for publication implies the transfer of the copyright from the author to the publisher upon acceptance. Accepted papers become the permanent property of 'Acta Haematologica' and may not be reproduced by any means, in whole or in part, without the written consent of the publisher. It is the author's responsibility to obtain permission to reproduce illustrations, tables, etc. from other publications.

## Arrangement

*Recommendation for Usage of Units and Abbreviations:* The Editorial Board of 'Acta Haematologica' supports the recommendations of the 'International Committee for Standardization in Hematology' for using the SI (Système International d'Unités) equivalents in haematological literature. The standard abbreviations used for measurements of weight, length, volume, and time (i.e. mg, cm, ml, min) are used without definition. The abbreviations listed on the opposite page also require no definition. Please note that punctuation is not needed. When using other abbreviations, spell out the name in full at the first mention, and follow with the abbreviation in parentheses.

*Title page:* The first page of each paper should indicate the title, the authors' names, and the institute where the work was conducted. A short title for use as running head as well as the full address of the author to whom correspondence should be sent are also required.

*Full address:* The exact postal address complete with postal code must be given at the bottom of the title page. Please also supply phone and fax numbers, as well as your e-mail address.

*Key words:* For indexing purposes, a list of 3–10 key words in English is essential.

*Abstract:* Each paper needs an abstract of up to 10 lines.

*Small type:* Paragraphs which can or must be set in smaller type (case histories, test methods, etc.) should be indicated with a 'p' (petit) in the margin on the left-hand side.

*Footnotes:* Avoid footnotes. When essential, they are numbered consecutively and typed at the foot of the appropriate page.

*Tables and illustrations:* Tables and illustrations (both numbered in Arabic numerals) should be prepared on separate sheets. Tables require a heading and figures a legend, also prepared on a separate sheet. For the reproduction of illustrations, only good drawings and original photographs can be accepted; negatives or photocopies cannot be used. Due to technical reasons, figures with a screen background should not be submitted. When possible, group several illustrations on one block for reproduction (max. size 180 × 223 mm) or provide crop marks. On the back of each illustration, indicate its number, the author's name, and 'top' with a soft pencil.

*Color illustrations:* Up to 6 color illustrations per page can be integrated within the text at the reduced price of CHF 660.–/USD 545.00 per page. Color illustrations are reproduced at the author's expense.

*References:* In the text identify references by Arabic numerals [in square brackets]. Material submitted for publication but not yet accepted should be noted as 'unpublished data' and not be included in the reference list. The list of references should include only those publications which are cited in the text. Do not alphabetize; number references in the order in which they are first mentioned in the text. The surnames of the authors followed by initials should be given. There should be no punctuation other than a comma to separate the authors. Cite all authors, 'et al' is not sufficient. Abbreviate journal names according to the Index Medicus system. (Also see International Committee of Medical Journal Editors: Uniform requirements for manuscripts submitted to biomedical journals. N Engl J Med 1997;336:309–315.)

*Examples*

*(a) Papers published in periodicals:* Sun J, Koto H, Chung KF: Interaction of ozone and allergen challenges on bronchial responsiveness and inflammation in sensitised guinea pigs. Int Arch Allergy Immunol 1997;112:191–195.

*(b) Monographs:* Matthews DE, Farewell VT: Using and Understanding Medical Statistics, ed 3, revised. Basel, Karger, 1996.

*(c) Edited books:* Parren PWHI, Burton DR: Antibodies against HIV-1 from phage display libraries: Mapping of an immune response and progress towards antiviral immunotherapy; in Capra JD (ed): Antibody Engineering. Chem Immunol. Basel, Karger, 1997, vol 65, pp 18–56.

## Page Charges

Authors are charged CHF 138.–/USD 98.00 per printed page for the first 6 pages and CHF 275.–/USD 196.00 for each additional page, including tables, illustrations, and references. 1 printed page is equal to approximately 3 manuscript pages.

## Rapid Communication

Manuscripts intended for rapid communication must present new findings of sufficient importance to justify their accelerated acceptance. They should follow the general arrangement of research papers except that the separate sections should not be formally titled. They should not be more than three pages in length (including figures, tables and references). Proofs are checked by the Main Editor and not sent to the authors. Review will be rapid, and once accepted, the paper will be included in the next planned issue. If manuscripts require significant change after editing they will be treated as brief communications and returned to the authors for correction.

## Brief Communication

The general arrangement for brief communications is the same as for research papers except that the manuscript is not divided into separate sections formally entitled introduction, methods, results, discussion. No abstract is required. These should not be more than 3 pages in length.

## Letter to the Editor

Comments and responses to previously published articles and other short correspondences are welcome. They should be limited to 1 or 1 1/2 manuscript pages with a general arrangement as specified for Brief Communications.

## Galley Proofs

Unless indicated otherwise, galley proofs are sent to the first-named author and should be returned with the least possible delay. Alterations made in galley proofs, other than the correction of printer's errors, are charged to the author. No page proofs are supplied.

## Reprints

Order forms and a price list are sent with the galley proofs. Orders submitted after the issue is printed are subject to considerably higher prices.

KARGER

Fax +41 61 306 12 34
E-Mail karger@karger.ch
www.karger.com



The Guidelines for Authors are available at:
www.karger.com/journals/aha/aha_gl.htm

# General Information

*Acta Hæmatologica*

**Publication data:** 'Acta Haematologica' is published 8 times a year. Volumes 103, 104 with 4 issues each appear in 2000.

**Subscription rates:** Subscriptions run for a full calendar year. Prices are given per volume.
*Personal subscription:*
*Subscription + postage and handling*
CHF 276.– + CHF 17.30 Europe
CHF 276.– + CHF 26.10 Overseas
USD 211.00 + USD 17.30
+ online subscription per volume:
CHF 39.–/USD 30.00
(Must be in the name of, billed to, and paid by an individual. Order must be marked 'personal subscription'.)
*Institutional subscription:*
*Subscription + postage and handling*
CHF 552.– + CHF 21.60 Europe
CHF 552.– + CHF 32.60 Overseas
USD 422.00 + USD 21.60
+ online subscription per volume:
CHF 58.–/USD 45.00
*Airmail postage:* CHF 24.–, USD 20.00.
(Extra per volume.)
*Discount subscription prices:*
International Society of Haematology

**Microforms:** Please direct all enquiries and orders to: University Microfilms Inc.
300 North Zeeb Road, P.O. Box 1346
Ann Arbor, MI 48106-1346 (USA)

**Subscription orders:** Orders can be placed at agencies, bookstores, directly with the Publisher
S. Karger AG, P.O. Box,
CH–4009 Basel (Switzerland)
or with any of the following distributors:
*Deutschland:* S. Karger GmbH, Postfach
D–79095 Freiburg
*France:* Librairie Luginbühl
36, bd de Latour-Maubourg, F–75007 Paris
*Great Britain, Ireland:* S. Karger Publishers
58 Grove Hill Road
Tunbridge Wells, Kent TN1 1SP
*USA:* S. Karger Publishers, Inc.
26 West Avon Road, P.O. Box 529
Farmington, CT 06085
*India, Bangladesh, Sri Lanka:*
S. Karger India Subscription Agency
B–5/132 Safdarjung Enclave
New Delhi-110029
*Japan:* Katakura Libri, Inc.
2F, Marushima Bldg, 4-6-17, Yushima,
Bunkyo-ku, Tokyo 113-0034

**Change of address:** Both old and new address should be sent to the subscription source.

**Single issues and back volumes:** Information can be obtained through the Publisher.

**Advertising:** Correspondence and rate requests should be addressed to the Publisher.

**Bibliographic indices:** This journal is regularly listed in bibliographic services, including *Current Contents®*.

**Book Reviews:** Books are accepted for review by special agreement.



## Usage of Units and Abbreviations

| Entity | Abbreviation | Recommended SI equivalent | Not recommended |
|---|---|---|---|
| Red blood cell count | RBC | $10^{12}$/l | $10^6$/mm$^3$ |
| White blood cell count | WBC | $10^9$/l | $10^3$/mm$^3$ |
| Platelet count | | ... × $10^9$/l | ... × $10^3$/mm$^3$ |
| Reticulocyte count | | % (or ... × $10^9$/l) | % (or ../mm$^3$) |
| Haemoglobin | Hb | g/dl[a] | g/100 ml |
| Packed cell volume | PCV | ratio[b] | % |
| Mean cell volume | MCV | fl | |
| Mean cell haemoglobin | MCH | pg | |
| Mean cell haemoglobin concentration | MCHC | g/dl | % |
| Mean cell diameter | MCD | μm | |
| Sedimentation rate | ESR | mm in 1 h[c] | |
| Plasma haemoglobin | Plasma Hb | mg/l | mg/100 ml |
| Serum vitamin $B_{12}$ | | ng/l | |
| Serum folate | | μg/l | |
| Serum iron | | μmol/l | μg/100 ml |
| Total iron binding capacity | TIBC | μmol/l | μg/100 ml |
| Unsaturated iron binding capacity | UIBC | μmol/l | μg/100 ml |
| Transferrin | | g/l | mg/100 ml |
| Serum haptoglobin | | g/l | mg/100 ml |
| Plasma fibrinogen | | g/l | mg/100 ml |

a The concentration for Hb only is expressed as ../dl and not ../l or ../100 ml.
b No unit necessary, 1/1 is implied.
c Indicate method only if other than Westergren.

KARGER

Fax +41 61 306 12 34
E-Mail karger@karger.ch
www.karger.com



The Journal Home Page is available at:
www.karger.com/journals/aha

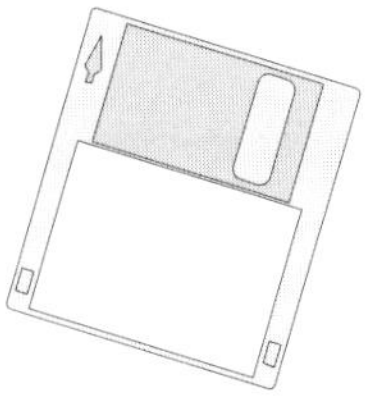

## Disk Submission

A **comprehensive version** of these guidelines for the **submission of manuscripts and illustrations on disk** can be accessed online under **www.karger.com/journals/disksub.htm** or requested as a leaflet from the editorial department.

Please follow the general rules on style and arrangement in the **'Guidelines for Authors'** of the journal. Submit a **double-spaced printout** of your manuscript matching the file on disk exactly.

**Technical Information**
Store only data pertinent to this manuscript. Include your fonts (screen and printer fonts for Macintosh). For a **text only** manuscript, use a 3.5-inch disk. For **text and illustrations,** use 3.5 or 5.25 Magneto Optical Disc; CD-ROM (DOS or hybrid); iomage Zip/DOS (100 MB), or 44 MB, 88 MB or 200 MB SyQuest. Compress extensive data using ZIP format.

**Data Description**
**Label** your disk with the **title of the journal or book** for which it is submitted; a **short version** of the paper's title; your **name,** postal and e-mail address, fax and phone number; **hard and software** used, including the version; and the **complete list of the file names.** File names consist of eight characters before the dot identifying the file and three characters after the dot identifying the application.

**Text and Format**
The **preferred word-processing package is MS-Word.** Other commonly used PC text programs and ASCII formats are accepted.
**Update your data** when you revise subsequent to the reviewer's or editor's decision and mark revisions clearly. Manuscripts accepted for publication are subject to **copy editing:** changes and/or questions will be marked in the manuscript, which will be returned to you with your disk and the galley proofs for checking.
**Enter your text continuously flush left.** Do not use any layout functions. Do not split words at the end of a line. **Do not use indentations.** Use a blank line before and a hard return at the end of paragraphs.
**Arrange headings flush left.** Insert only **one space after punctuation marks.** Insert Greek letters, mathematical symbols etc. with your word-processing program. Use **boldface and italics** as well as sub- and superscript where appropriate.
**Tables are part of the text** and should be placed at the end of the text file. Separate the individual parts of a table by lines. Use the tabulator instead of spaces. Format operation data on one line in the same column. **Legends to illustrations are part of the text** and should also be listed at the end of the text file.

**Illustrations**
**Store illustrations as separate files:** do not integrate them in your text. Export **line drawings/vector graphics** as TIF, EPS or WMF format. Use Photoshop for processing and retouching **scanned halftone images.** Save the original scan and the processed version. Export **black and white or color images** as TIF or EPS format in their anticipated size in print.
**For detailed information** on how to submit illustration data on disk please consult the leaflet or **www.karger.com/journals/disksub.htm.**

KI 98 DISK




KARGER

Fax +41 61 306 12 34
E-Mail karger@karger.ch
www.karger.com





The Journal Home Page is available at:
www.karger.com/journals/aha

Acta Hæmatologica

# Is There a Cure for Aplastic Anaemia?

In memoriam Bruno Speck
1934–1998

Editor
*Catherine Nissen,* Basel

15 figures and 19 tables, 2000

KARGER

Basel · Freiburg · Paris · London · New York ·
New Delhi · Bangkok · Singapore · Tokyo · Sydney

S. Karger
Medical and Scientific Publishers
Basel · Freiburg · Paris · London
New York · New Delhi · Bangkok
Singapore · Tokyo · Sydney

Drug Dosage
The authors and the publisher have exerted every effort to ensure that drug selection and dosage set forth in this text are in accord with current recommendations and practice at the time of publication. However, in view of ongoing research, changes in government regulations, and the constant flow of information relating to drug therapy and drug reactions, the reader is urged to check the package insert for each drug for any change in indications and dosage and for added warnings and precautions. This is particularly important when the recommended agent is a new and/or infrequently employed drug.


Printed in Switzerland on acid-free paper by
Reinhardt Druck, Basel
ISBN 3–8055–7040–6

KARGER

Fax+ 41 61 306 12 34
E-Mail karger@karger.ch
www.karger.com

Acta Hæmatologica

# Contents Vol. 103, No. 1, 2000



KARGER

Fax+ 41 61 306 12 34
E-Mail karger@karger.ch
www.karger.com



Access to full text and tables of contents,
including tentative ones for forthcoming issues:
www.karger.com/journals/aha/aha_bk.htm

Acta Haematologica

Acta Haematol 2000;103:4

# Preface

This special issue of *Acta Haematologica* is dedicated to Bruno Speck, a pioneer in the treatment of severe aplastic anaemia (SAA). His major contributions were the detection of a link between SAA and exposure to chloramphenicol together with Sven Moeschlin and the introduction of antilymphocyte globulin (ALG) for the treatment of SAA patients not eligible for stem cell transplantation. His aim was to improve the prognosis of SAA: scientific success was secondary. Many of his patients remember him as a caring doctor. Having shared the joy of seeing the first SAA patients recover after ALG, we also witnessed Bruno Speck's disappointment when trying to convince the professional world that ALG is effective in SAA.

The originality of Bruno Speck's experimental work was recognised early in *Acta Haematologica*, where results of preclinical ALG studies [1973;50:193–199] and the first positive clinical results [1976;55:129–139] were published. It took 10 more years before ALG/ATG became standard treatment. That ALG – in contrast to stem cell transplantation – does not cure SAA became apparent with long-term observations. This does not lessen the value of ALG/ATG: it is often lifesaving as first-line treatment, as illustrated by a case report included in this issue.

The following articles are personally dedicated to Bruno Speck by his colleagues, collaborators and one of his patients, who have followed the 'ALG story' from its beginnings to its success. Apart from giving an update on the state of the art, the contributions are a homage to Bruno, who was an original clinical researcher in haematology, an excellent teacher and a dear friend. In addition, they may trigger further research aiming at the improvement of treatment outcomes of patients with SAA, or at preventing the disease. This could be a wish of Bruno Speck, who left us too early.

*Catherine Nissen*, Basel

KARGER

Fax + 41 61 306 12 34
E-Mail karger@karger.ch
www.karger.com



Accessible online at:
www.karger.com/journals/aha

Acta Hæmatologica

Acta Haematol 2000;103:5–6

# Remembering Bruno Speck

The death of Bruno Speck in September of 1998 leaves all of us in the bone marrow transplant field saddened. We have lost a friend and colleague and will miss his presence dearly.

Bruno began his career in bone marrow transplantation in 1969 in Leiden, Holland, where he began a close and lasting friendship with Jon van Rood. He helped found the bone marrow transplantation program in Leiden. Among other accomplishments at Leiden, he was lead author on a manuscript in 1973 describing the first attempt to treat aplastic anemia with bone marrow from a phenotypically matched unrelated donor. While at Leiden he also became interested in the observations of George Mathé that some patients given antilymphocyte globulin and bone marrow infusions improved even though engraftment was transient or not evident. Over the next decade, his laboratory and clinical work established immunosuppression with ATG as an effective treatment for patients with aplastic anemia and this has become a standard alternative to bone marrow transplantation for this disease. Bruno also developed the rabbit as a successful animal model for studying the pathogenesis of aplastic anemia and subsequently his laboratory utilized the rabbit model for other transplantation studies. In 1980, Bruno received the Ernst Jung Award for Medicine for his basic studies on the pathogenesis and treatment of aplastic anemia.

Bruno returned to Switzerland in 1973 to establish one of the first bone marrow transplantation programs in the world in Basel. In addition to his work on aplastic anemia, his program became one of the first to treat leukemia successfully with bone marrow transplantation. The Basel group were among the pioneers who treated patients with chronic myeloid leukemia in the chronic phase with bone marrow transplantation and who, along with investigators at the Royal Marsden Hospital in London, evaluated cyclosporin for the treatment and prevention of graft-versus-host disease.

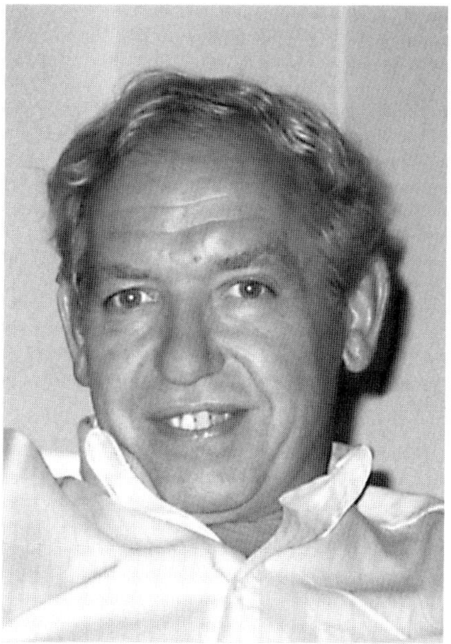

Bruno Speck (1934–1998).

One of the major achievements of Bruno Speck was his understanding that progress in bone marrow transplanta-

KARGER

Fax + 41 61 306 12 34
E-Mail karger@karger.ch
www.karger.com



Accessible online at:
www.karger.com/journals/aha

tion could only be achieved by mutual collaboration. To this end, it was his philosophy and that of Jon van Rood that created the European Group for Blood and Marrow Transplantation (EBMT). He and Jon organized a meeting of active investigators of EBMT (Drs. van Rood, Gluckman, Bussel, Zwaan, Vossen and Cornu) in St. Moritz in 1975. This meeting led to the establishment of the EBMT which has become a major force in the bone marrow transplantation field. The EBMT now includes over 2,500 members and is a tribute to Bruno's foresight.

As Director of Hematology, Kantonsspital Basel, since 1979, Bruno was also responsible for day-to-day activities of a large hematology department. He was esteemed by all of his colleagues and trained a number of investigators, teachers and practitioners throughout Switzerland and the world. All of us who have known Bruno will remember him not only for his skills as a clinician and researcher but also for his warm personality and his positive attitude to life. We all owe a lot to Bruno.

*C. Dean Buckner,* MD, Seattle, Wash.

Acta Hæmatologica

Acta Haematol 2000;103:7–10

# Bruno Speck in Leiden: The Clinician, the Scientist, the Man

Bruno's arrival in Leiden was memorable. It was March 30 1969, a cloudy and cold day with a light drizzle; typical 'Dutch weather' for those who do not live in Holland. Bruno arrived in his Porsche, enthusiastically explaining how safe it was to drive 180 km/h in bad weather conditions as long as you did it in a Porsche. He loved that car. I had been waiting for him at the entrance of the Isolation Pavilion, his future place of work. The Isolation Pavilion had been built by the Institute for the protection and treatment of radiation accident victims. It was quite new and had four isolation rooms, a novelty in those days. Fortunately, there had not yet been any radiation accidents and the unit had been used for the treatment of patients with aplastic anemia and leukemia, those receiving a kidney transplant, and one child with severe combined immunodeficiency who was unsuccessfully transplanted with bone marrow cells from an unrelated donor.

The University Hospital in Leiden was in the middle of a burst of activity in many fields, especially those concerning coagulation, immunohematology, blood transfusion and transplantation. This was an ideal playground for a young, enthusiastic and ambitious young clinician like Bruno.

## Bruno, the Clinician

We badly needed someone like Bruno. Oncohematology was almost nonexistent in Leiden; a surgeon with an interest in oncology was treating the Hodgkin's patients. Bruno fitted the bill to perfection. He had studied medicine in Bern (1952–1960), wrote his 'Doktorarbeit' on coagulation in 1961, had been a rotating intern in Seattle (1961–1962) and resident in Internal Medicine in the Mayo Clinics (1962–1965), with hematology as a subspecialization. Thereafter he returned to Switzerland where he worked in Solothurn with Professor Sven Moeschlin, a well-known Swiss hematologist. He had applied for the job in Leiden because of an advertisement in the 'Schweizerische Ärztezeitung'. Fredi Loeliger, who was in charge of the coagulation laboratory and himself a Swiss, contacted Moeschlin, received very favorable information, and Bruno was appointed as 'Wetenschappelijk Hoofdambtenaar A', a position equivalent to an associate professorship nowadays. His tasks were to run the Isolation Pavilion, to take over the responsibility for the treatment of oncohematological patients outside the Isolation Pavilion, to do research, and to teach.

Leiden was in a very favorable position to intensify the treatment of oncohematological and aplastic patients. The discovery that antibodies were formed during pregnancy, recognizing what later turned out to be the human lymphocyte antigen (HLA) system, and the unraveling of the genetic complexity of HLA by computer-supported statistical analysis made it possible to assess the clinical relevance of HLA. It could indeed be shown that HLA matching improved the effectiveness of platelet and granulocyte transfusions and improved renal allograft survival. The first successful HLA identical sibling bone marrow transplant in Europe, in a 4-month-old patient with severe

KARGER

Fax + 41 61 306 12 34
E-Mail karger@karger.ch
www.karger.com



Accessible online at:
www.karger.com/journals/aha

combined immune deficiency, had been performed in the pediatric department in Leiden, six months before Bruno's arrival and almost at the same time as those in the United States.

The close collaboration with Dick van Bekkum and his coworkers in the Radio Biological Institute (Rijswijk) should be mentioned in this context. They had developed a stem cell transplant model, first in the mouse and later in primates, and were actively involved in the clinical application of bone marrow transplantation. They had also developed a reversed isolation protocol to protect the (decontaminated) patient from outside pathogens, which was introduced in the Leiden pediatric department, but rarely used elsewhere. This was in itself a pity, because it has been shown that the procedure, costly and labor-intensive as it is, diminishes graft versus host disease (GVHD).

Bruno learned to speak Dutch (essential for the contact with patients) in a few months and even before that time was able to interact directly with the patients. He was a born clinician: solid and trust inspiring. The patients loved him. Fortunately, he liked teaching and was very good at it, both at the bedside and during 'grand rounds'. He was also able to absorb and integrate new information quickly and soon learned when HLA was useful in the clinic and when not. In later years, he often thanked me that he had learned so much from us. I always thought it was the other way around.

He reorganized the procedures in the Isolation Pavilion right away. A few adult patients had been unsuccessfully transplanted with bone marrow from related and unrelated donors before his arrival. This experience formed the basis for a detailed protocol for the treatment of aplastic anemia (SAA) and leukemia. There was a renewed interest in SAA, not only because of the pioneering work of Don Thomas (Seattle) and colleagues, but especially because of the observation of George Mathé, Schwarzenberg and Amiel (Paris) that conditioning of the patient with ATG, followed by a bone marrow transplantation, could apparently cure SAA without the risk of GVHD. There was interest but also a lot of scepticism. To resolve the debate over whether or not true chimerism existed, a round table discussion was organized in Munich, where Amiel defended the position of the French that chimerism indeed existed.

The sceptics were clearly in the majority, however, and after 40 min of intensive debate, Amiel, an awfully nice person, but probably the most ugly man I have ever met, threw his arms in the air and cried in true Anglo-French: 'I am like the most beautiful girl on earth; I cannot give more than I 'ave', and sat down. Bruno also did not convince the audience.

From the beginning, we were believers for no good reason other than that it appeared to work in Paris, and the first SAA patient was treated unsuccessfully with antilymphocyte globulin (ALG) and bone marrow shortly after Bruno's arrival. It would take until 1974 before the treatment (ALG plus bone marrow from the father!) was successfully carried out in a 14-year-old girl.

Bruno also updated the treatment of leukemia. Daunorubicin and arabinoside-cytoline were introduced, and the first 'complete' remissions in acute leukemia patients were achieved, a breakthrough from the 6-mercaptopurine-prednisone regimes. Bone marrow transplantation for acute leukemia was also attempted but was unsuccessful.

Every Tuesday afternoon, the hematology rounds took place. Not only SAA and leukemia patients, but also patients with coagulation disorders, acquired and congenital hemolytic anemia, and thrombocytopenia were reviewed. The Leiden hematology department existed! It was an exciting time. Bob Epstein, trained by Don Thomas, was a visiting Boerhaave Professor and provided advice from his experience in Seattle. An attempt to copy the Seattle dog model in Leiden was unfortunately unsuccessful.

Bruno's activities were also instrumental in introducing cytogenetics into the clinic, and in the recognition of the first patient with hairy cell leukemia in Leiden [1].

He was a good morphologist and could and would argue with Paul Lopes Cardozo, who was running the hematomorphology and cytology laboratories.

Several residents, such as Hans Haak, Martin Fickers, Ferry Zwaan and others, worked with Bruno in the Isolation Pavilion and elsewhere. It speaks for his enthusiasm and teaching abilities that many of them retained their interest in hematology.

After his departure to Basel, we remained in close contact and consulted with each other about difficult patients. It was only after a long telephone conversation in 1975 that we decided to treat an SAA patient with ATG only. That patient recovered.

## Bruno, the Scientist

When applying for the job in Leiden, Bruno also submitted a list of his publications up to that point (table 1). He had been working with Moeschlin on an experimental model of SAA induced by benzene in rabbits (table 1: 4, 6,

**Table 1.** List of publications submitted by Bruno Speck when applying for the job in Leiden

| | |
|---|---|
| 1. | Doktorarbeit Universität Bern 1961 |
| 2. | Thesis M.S., University of Minnesota Graduate School |
| 3. | The significance of autoantibodies. In: Seminars in Medicine and Physiology at the Mayo Graduate School 101 – 113, 1964/65. |
| 4. | Experimentelle Untersuchungen über den Wirkungsmechanismus des Benzols auf das Knochenmark. Autoradiographische Untersuchungen mit H-Thymidin, Schweiz. Med. Wschr. 96:74–76, 1966. |
| 5. | Failure of L-phenylalanine to prevent benzene induced pancytopenia. Experientia 23: 481–484, 1967. |
| 6. | Experimental studies on the mechanism of action of benzene on the bone marrow (Radioautographic studies using $^3$H-Thymidine). Acta Haematologica 38:104–111, 1967. |
| 7. | Die diurnale Schwankung des Serumeisens und der latenten Eisenbindungskapazität beim normalen Erwachsenen. Helv. Med. Acta Suppl. 47:140, 1967. |
| 8. | Hematopoietic effects of a folate antagonist in man. Cancer 20:225–232, 1967. |
| 9. | Klinische Prüfung des Gastrotherapeuticum Aluten. Praxis 56:1502–1504, 1967. |
| 10. | The diurnal variation of the serum iron and of the latent iron-binding capacity in normal adults. Helv. Med. Acta (1968 im Druck). |
| 11. | Untersuchungen der Nierenfunktion mit radioaktivem Diatrirost und o-Jodhippursäure (Schweiz. Internisten-Kongress, Chur 1968). |
| 12. | Autoradiographische Untersuchungen über die Wirkung verschiedener myelotoxischer Substanzen auf das Knochenmark (Schweiz. Hämatologenkongress, Chur 1968). |

12). Aware of Mathé's attempts to treat SAA by bone marrow transplantation and ATG, he quickly realized that his benzene-rabbit model would offer an ideal opportunity to asses the relevance of Mathé's observations. To say that he realized his opportunity is an understatement; he was completely engrossed by it.

Shortly after his arrival, I took him on a sailing trip on the Rhine and through the Biesbosch, one of the most beautiful and interesting Dutch water landscapes. When I pointed out to him a particularly nice scene, Bruno looked up vaguely and murmured: 'I need 14 rabbits at least to start off with'. I must confess that I was slightly irritated. Work is indeed important, but it should not interfere with sailing and the enjoyment of it!

Anyhow, I agreed with the importance of his protocol, and soon the Isolation Pavilion had two nursing areas: the patients inside and the rabbits outside. Margot Kissling, Bruno's dedicated technician, was taking care of the experimental protocol, and their first publication from Leiden appeared in 1971 [2]. Probably because it was published in French, and only shortly after the publication of the study by Amiel et al. [3] showing the effectiveness of this protocol in humans, it did not receive the recognition it deserved. Although disappointed, Bruno and Margot Kissling continued to work on that protocol. It took until 1973 before they were widely quoted [4].

One of our best technicians, Henriette Goselink, joined them and helped to set up the in vitro tests, such as colony-forming units tests, necessary to study the fate of the grafts. She recalls that this was not always easy. Margot Kissling and Bruno communicated in rapid 'Schwizerdüütsch', and although it sounds a bit like Dutch, many words have a different meaning.

The animal facilities were decidedly primitive, and Bruno, together with Cor Martijn, the caretaker of the animals, handyman and laboratory assistant, decided to upgrade the stable. The rabbit facility was modernized, including a system of collecting and flushing away the feces and urine via a wide gutter placed under the cages. The rabbits did not like it, developed cystitis and hand cleaning was reinstated.

## Bruno, the Man

Moeschlin had wholeheartedly recommended Bruno as a levelheaded, good physician with a real interest in preclinical models for the study of SAA. He noted also that Bruno was 'ein lieber Mensch' (a nice guy) who was still slightly naïve. It typifies Bruno exactly.

He was always pleasant and steady. I cannot remember having ever seen him really angry, although he certainly was disappointed that his ideas on SAA and ATG had not received international recognition at that time. That did not mean to say that he could not give good guidance to his staff. He treated them as equals and gave them full responsibility. If he did not get his way, he had an effective alternative: he just looked miserable.

Hans Haak remembers that he almost missed the birth of his second child, because it coincided with a bone marrow harvest and Bruno had looked so unhappy that Haak had given in. On the other hand, Bruno was also greatly appreciated, because he not only treated his staff as equals but also helped them with whatever had to be done if there were not enough hands available.

He loved a good party and was fond of a good glass of whiskey. There was always a bottle in his room and after hours (and against the rules) those still present would join

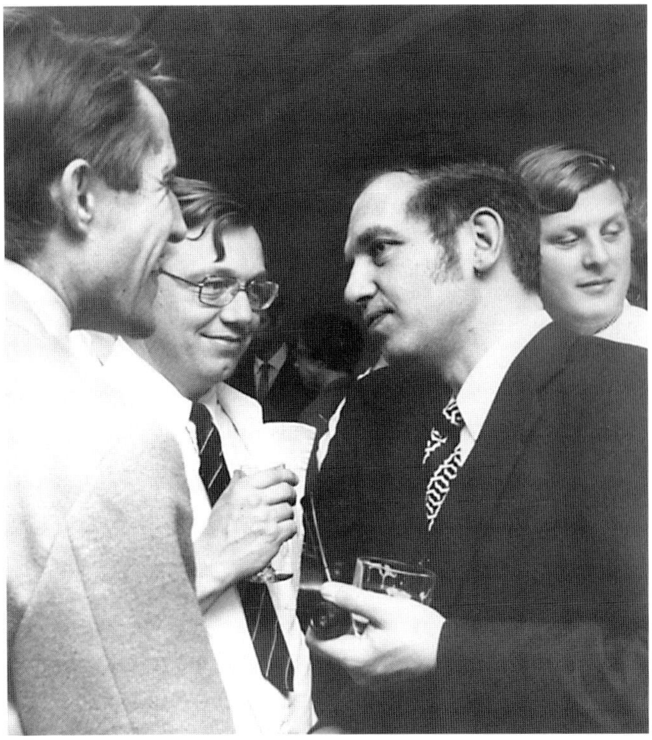

**Fig. 1.** An after-hours chat (and drink) with Jan Veltkamp and Ferry Zwaan.

him for a drink (fig. 1). On one occasion, the caretaker of the animals, Cor Martijn, had to work through the weekend, felt sorry for himself and finished the bottle. The next day, Bruno looked quizzical but said nothing. The following day, he came back with two bottles of whiskey, gave one to Cor Martijn and told him: 'This bottle is yours and this one is mine and you keep your hands off it'. No wonder his staff liked him so much!

It was precisely this charm that was so effective in starting what would later become the EBMT. The year was 1973, the year Bruno left us. Bone marrow transplantation was carried out by a handful of centers in Europe: by Eliane Gluckman in Paris; by Ted Gordon-Smith, John Barret, John Goldman and John Hobbs in London; in Leiden, Basel and a few other places. The results were appalling.

We came together for a symposium in Frankfurt, and in the evening visited a 'Bierkeller' to discuss our problems further. At the end, I went to the podium to summarize the discussions. I noted that the results were disappointing and that collaboration was essential. I concluded by saying that we had the choice either to join forces and develop a European protocol or to leave it up to Seattle. Seattle did that anyhow, but it was decided there to come together in the spring of 1974 to discuss the clinical results and protocols. Bruno offered to organize the first meeting in St. Moritz and, assisted by Pierre Cornu and other members of his staff, did so to perfection. In the context of this chapter, the importance of the EBMT for Europe and bone marrow transplantation does not need further explanation.

The impact of Bruno's scientific work and his personality on the development of hematology in Europe and throughout the world cannot be overestimated.

Prof. Dr. *J.J. van Rood*, Leiden


**Acknowledgements**

I would like to thank Fredi Loeliger, Henriette Goselink, Hans Haak, Martin Fickers and Leo Jan Dooren for reading the manuscript and providing anecdotes which bring Bruno's presence in Leiden so much in focus again.


**References**


1 Haak HL, de Man JC, Hijmans W, Speck B: Further evidence for the lymphocytic nature of leukaemic reticuloendotheliosis (hairy-cell leukaemia). Br J Haematol 1974;27:31–38.
2 Speck B, Kissling M: Successful bone marrow grafts in experimental aplastic anemia using antilymphocytic serum for conditioning. Rev Eur Etud Clin Biol 1971;16:1047–1051.
3 Amiel JL, Mathé G, Schwarzenberg L, Schneider M, Choay J, Trolard P, Hayat M, Schlumberger JR, Jasmin C: Allogenic bone marrow graft after conditioning with only antilymphocytic serum in states of bone marrow aplasias (in French). Presse Méd 1970;78: 1727–1734.
4 Speck B, Kissling M: Studies on bone marrow transplantation in experimental $^{32}$P-induced aplastic anemia after conditioning with antilymphocyte serum. Acta Haematol 1973;50: 193–199.

Acta Hæmatologica

Acta Haematol 2000;103:11–15

# Aplastic Anemia before Bone Marrow Transplantation and Antilymphocyte Globulin

Hermann Heimpel

Medizinische Universitätsklinik, Ulm, Deutschland

**Key Words**

Aplastic anemia · Prognostic factor · Secondary leukemia

**Abstract**

In severe aplastic anemia, disease-dependent mortality was high before allogeneic bone marrow transplantation (BMT) and immunosuppressive therapies (IST) including antilymphocyte globulin became available. However, under supportive therapy alone, spontaneous remissions were observed in up to 20% of severe cases, reflecting the natural course of the disease. Therefore, in evaluating new forms of treatment, one has to keep in mind that remission is not necessarily response, and that final proof of utility of any new therapy still requires a randomized study design. Transition to leukemia or myelodysplasia was rarely observed if the initial diagnosis was accurate. The much higher incidence of leukemias in patients treated by IST, but not by BMT is probably due to the better life expectancy of patients at risk, rather than to a leukemogenic potential of IST itself. 'Outdated' therapeutic modalities, such as androgens or splenectomy, may still be justified as an adjuvant therapy in selected cases.



In clinical medicine, and particularly in hematology, the success of a novel therapy is often the final proof of a pathophysiological hypothesis which was based on in vitro studies and circumstantial evidence from clinical observation. Bruno Speck's work on the efficacy of antilymphocyte globulin (ALG) in severe aplastic anemia is a striking paradigm. Bruno was an open-minded researcher, who did not feel compelled to hide results of his work before publication. Because of this attitude, based on his conviction that the patient's good has priority over the acknowledgment of personal merits, I had knowledge of his early results even before their publication in the *Lancet* in 1977 [1]. He gave us ALG from his horse Volcano[1] to treat two patients with severe aplastic anemia. Treatment was followed by remission in one patient, but was ineffective in the other.

This issue in memory of Bruno Speck is an opportunity to give a short description of the situation before allogeneic bone marrow transplantation (BMT) and immunosuppression altered the natural course of the disease.

[1] Others claim that the horse's name was Caesar; in any case, it was a brave, immunocompetent horse!

KARGER

Fax + 41 61 306 12 34
E-Mail karger@karger.ch
www.karger.com


0001–5792/00/1031–0011$17.50/0

Accessible online at:
www.karger.com/journals/aha

Prof. Dr. med. H. Heimpel
Medizinische Universitätsklinik
Robert-Koch-Strasse 8
D–89081 Ulm (Germany)
E-Mail hermann.heimpel@medizin.uni-ulm.de

## Natural Course of Aplastic Anemia

Before the advent of allogeneic BMT and immunosuppressive therapy (IST), most patients with aplastic anemia died of the complications of their disease. Median survival was only 10 months in 101 cases of aplastic anemia of different severity followed by Williams et al. [2] from 1944 to 1973 and even less in other series reporting patients seen before 1970 [3]. Others [4, 5] have reported longer survival, but when these early reports are considered, one has to keep in mind that diagnostic criteria where not well defined. Analysis of bone marrow often relied on aspiration cytology alone; hence pancytopenias of other origin, such as hairy cell leukemia, hypoplastic leukemia or refractory anemia were erroneously included. In later series, early mortality was reduced by the improvements of supportive therapy, platelet transfusions and bactericidal antibiotics. In a retrospective study on our own 70 patients from 1967 to 1974 [6], median survival was 20 months for all, and only 10 months for patients with risk factors, a group defined by almost identical parameters as severe aplastic anemia according to Camitta et al. [7] in 1976. The poor prognosis in severely affected patients was still due to early mortality only in a minority; more significant was patients' refractoriness to platelet substitution resulting from long-standing irreversibility of aplasia, bleeding being responsible for the majority of deaths. Almost identical results were reported by others [8, 9], suggesting that low blood counts alone do not determine the acute risk, but rather reflect the degree of the underlying damage to the hemopoietic stem cell pool itself, or possibly the underlying pathophysiology in a pathophysiologically heterogeneous, albeit phenotypically similar disease. Further retrospective studies in the following years reported overall median survival times between 20 and 60 months. These large differences are most probably related to differences in patient selection, with aggregation of more serious cases in centers known for their interest in aplastic anemia [10].

Remissions, however, were observed in all groups, also including in the high-risk patients. In our extended survey of 113 patients with severe and nonsevere aplastic anemia, 47% reached partial or complete remission, with extended survival observed over 8 years [11]. In patients corresponding to the later definition of severe aplastic anemia, remissions were significantly less frequent at 16%, but there were no differences in late prognosis between patients with or without risk factors after complete or partial remission was reached. Similar rates of spontaneous remissions were seen by others. After remission, relapses were rarely observed. This is in sharp contrast to the situation of patients who had improved after IST [12], showing an actuarial relapse rate of 35% after 14 years. This observation, as well as the few prospective randomized trials of IST versus 'conventional therapy' with androgens or supportive care alone [13–15], can serve as a strong argument for the specific efficacy of IST. After spontaneous remission, blood and bone marrow may become completely normal, but as for remissions induced by IST, subnormal or borderline low leukocyte or platelet counts and red cell macrocytosis may persist for many years.

## Therapy-Independent Prognostic Factors

Prognostic factors were extensively studied before and after the availability of effective therapy. Only the former, or those obtained from control arms in prospective randomized studies, reflect biological differences of the underlying defect itself. All others also reflect the probability of response to a specific therapy such as in IST or the probability of therapy-related death following BMT. Therapy-independent prognostic factors were investigated in the hope of recognizing groups of heterogeneous origin, as well as to define subgroups used as historical controls and to select patients for allogeneic BMT, formerly a high-risk procedure. Acute onset [2, 5, 16] and male gender [2] were found to be negative prognostic factors, but correlations are too weak to be of actual relevance. Data on age were conflicting. Although bone marrow hypocellularity is one of the obligate definition criteria of aplastic anemia and is considered to reflect the fundamental functional defect in this disorder, the extent of of bone marrow hypocellularity does not correlate with prognosis. However, the intensity of the infiltrate by plasma cells and lymphocytes is clearly a negative prognostic factor [17–19]. These observations suggested that aplastic anemia of the autoimmune type may have a worse prognosis. This type of investigation, however, has not been repeated in patients treated by IST; hence, this hypothesis remains speculative.

Clearly, the most reliable prognostic factor is based on the most simple criterion, namely the severity of pancytopenia itself. There is no doubt that low counts of at least two of the three lineages affected are sufficient to define the subgroup of severe aplastic anemia with poor prognosis, regardless of the therapy chosen [6–9, 11, 20, 21]. Within this group, a low absolute reticulocyte count [22] and/or a neutrophil count of less then 200/μl suggest a particularly poor prognosis. However, some patients with transient pancytopenia may, for a short time, fulfill the criteria of severe aplastic anemia, and we have therefore advocated the use of counts obtained during a 3-month period to predict their chance of going into spontaneous remission. With today's capacity of early effective therapy, this suggestion is no longer valid, but one has to acknowledge that all series showing positive results contain some patients who would have spontaneously recovered with transient supportive treatment alone. In any case, decision-making should include evaluation of all blood counts available up to the time IST or conditioning for BMT begins, and it is still advisable to delay treatment if a clear upward trend of blood counts is observed.

Etiology was formerly regarded as relevant for prognosis. An association with exposure to chloramphenicol was regarded as a risk factor for both mortality and transition to leukemia. However, these data resulted from the uncritical analysis of case reports. More recent epidemiological data suggest a much lower fraction of drug-induced aplastic anemia than was formerly thought, and failed to detect a different response to therapy in cases suspected to be induced by drugs and those that were not [23]. Based on many case reports, aplastic anemia occurring in the course of viral hepatitis was regarded as having a particularly poor prognosis and therefore to be an indication for early BMT [24]. Whether this is still true with modern supportive care in the acute phase of the disorder is unknown. Patients may already improve during the time preparations for BMT are done, and others went into remission after IST [25].

### Differentiating between Chronic Aplastic Anemia and Transient Pancytopenia

Transient pancytopenia refers to an entity not generally recognized in the classification of hematological disorders. Cases of pancytopenia with a hypo- or normocellular bone marrow and spontaneous recovery within 10–90 days have been described as 'transitory bone marrow failure', 'transient aplastic anemia', 'bone marrow aplasia', 'bone marrow suppression' or 'reversible bone marrow aplasia' [for a review, see ref. 26]. Among cases of aplastic anemia, defined according to the criteria proposed by Heimpel and Kubaneck [27] and Camitta et al. [28], including bone marrow hypoplasia, 5% did not show a chronic course but fully recovered within 90 days, with most patients recovering within less than 1 month [26]. In other epidemiological studies, follow-up data are usually not available. Such series may contain cases of transient pancytopenia, particularly if reports on bone marrow biopsy are not required. In contrast, series devoted to therapy most probably include none or a very few such cases, which are often not referred to specialized research institutions. For the sake of drug safety and preventive measures in industrial hygiene or environmental policies, both conditions may be lumped together. This is not true when formulating working hypotheses of pathophysiology or assessing the efficacy of a specific therapy.

### Evolution of Aplastic Anemia to Leukemia and Myelodysplastic Syndromes

Patients progressing to acute myelogenous leukemia (AML) have been described since 1941, but in many reports data are incomplete and no clear distinction was made between true aplastic anemia and pancytopenia with nonhypoplastic bone marrow, now classified as myelodysplastic syndromes. It is the merit of Bruno Speck's group in Basel to have provided a detailed analysis of myelodysplasia or acute myeloid leukemia as late complications in patients who recovered from severe aplastic anemia after IST [29–31]. They have clearly shown that in patients treated by IST, but not by BMT, the relative risk of myelodysplastic syndrome (MDS)/AML is very high, and goes on increasing for more than 10 years after remission of aplastic anemia, with a probability of 26% after 15 years. Similar [32], but also lower probabilities [33] were seen by others. There are only a few data from the time before IST became available. Seven of 174 and 2 of 76 cases of leukemia after aplastic anemia were observed by Mir and Geary [9] and Gordon-Smith [34], respectively. In our series of 113 patients and a median observation time of 3 years, only 1 patient developed AML. No cases of leukemia or MDS were reported in the French series [8]. In summary, MDS/AML seems to be a potential late complication of aplastic anemia independent of IST. However, the paucity of older data does not allow one to finally decide whether the exceptionally high risk in the Basel series is due to the improved survival of high-risk patients alone, which reveals the natural evolution of severe cases, or whether IST as such is an additional risk factor. Dyshemopoietic morphological changes of hemopoietic cells in the marrow at the time of diagnosis and/or IST-induced recovery were more prominent in the Swiss cases who later developed MDS [30, 31]. A review of cases from many centers notified in the International Study on Agranulocytosis and

Aplastic Anemia has shown that the classification of such cases as aplastic anemia or hypoplastic MDS may be controversial [35]. We have also observed IST-induced remission in such borderline cases. The observation that partial or even complete remissions can be reached in these cases has prompted trials of IST in low-risk MDS.

## Other Modalities of Therapy besides ATG/Cyclosporin or Allogeneic BMT

Early attempts of pharmacotherapy were aimed at stimulating, directly or indirectly, the inadequate production of blood cells, based on the hypoplasia of the morphologically identifiable hemopoietic cells and their committed colony-forming precursors. Trials included a variety of drugs which lead to increased cell production in laboratory animals or humans. Apparent successes in single cases could not be confirmed by others, and were most probably due to spontaneous recovery in reversible aplastic anemia or transient pancytopenia [36]. One exception are androgens and their synthetic analogues. After early positive reports in both children [37] and adults [4], many phase-2 and a few randomized studies were performed. In the latter, no positive effect on survival or remission rates could be demonstrated [38–40]. The same is true for some [41, 42], but not all [43] studies testing the additional effect of androgens to IST. However, improved survival as compared to historical controls in some series including nonsevere cases [44, 45] and the observation of androgen dependency in single cases [36, 46] suggest that androgens can lead to some improvement in a minority of less severe [47] cases. Based on these observations, a trial of mesterelon or oxymethenolone is still justified in patients with nonsevere aplastic anemia or with partial remission, but insufficient recovery, in order to try and improve their quality of life compromised by anemia, or to lower the frequency of red cell transfusions.

Splenectomy was one of the modalities frequently tried even earlier, before androgens were used. Partial and complete remissions were reported in more than half of the patients [48–50, for a review, see 51]. From the data available, it seems that these were cases of nonsevere aplastic anemia, and since the diagnosis was usually based on bone marrow aspiration alone, these old series probably included other conditions responding to splenectomy, such as aleukemic hairy cell leukemia. However, some cases in which splenectomy was successful are well documented. We have also seen selected cases of nonsevere aplastic anemia where blood counts partially improved and transfusion dependency decreased after the spleen was removed. Again, it was the Basel group who systematically tested splenectomy as an adjuvant measure to treatment by ATG [52] and I fully agree with their statement that 'splenectomy should be reconsidered in selective nontransplanted patients who have prolonged transfusion requirements despite otherwise optimal treatment'.

## Conclusions

A look back to the situation of patients with aplastic anemia before effective IST was introduced by Bruno Speck and his group spotlights his merits as a research-oriented physician. Immune or even autoimmune reactions were suspected long ago as potential mechanisms of bone marrow failure [27, 51, 53]. Early attempts to test this hypothesis by IST were not convincing. In 1967, we had seen a complete remission in close temporal relationship to IST by azathioprine in a child with severe aplastic anemia not responding to androgens [54]. However, after similar trials in 11 further patients had failed, we abandoned this track. Bruno Speck, fortunately, but even more as a consequence of his scientific belief, found it.

## References


1 Speck B, Gluckman E, Haak HL, et al: Treatment of aplastic anaemia by antilymphocyte globulin with and without allogeneic bone-marrow infusions. Lancet 1977;ii:1145–1148.

2 Williams DM, Lynch RE, Cartwright GE: Prognostic factors in aplastic anemia. Clin Haematol 1978;7:467-474.

3 Davis S, Ruben AD: Treatment and prognosis of aplastic anemia. Lancet 1972;i:871.

4 Sanchez Medal L, Gomez Leal A, Duarte L, et al: Anabolic androgenic steroids in the treatment of acquired aplastic anemia. Blood 1969; 34:283–300.

5 Najean Y, Bernard J, Wainberger M, et al: Evolution et pronostic de pancytopenies idiopathiques. Etude de 116 observations. Nouv Rev Fr Hématol 1965;5:639–656.

6 Heimpel H, Rehbock C, Van Eimeren W: Verlauf und Prognose der Panmyelopathie und der isolierten aplastischen Anämie: Eine retrospective Studie an 70 Patienten. Blut 1975;30: 235–254.

7 Camitta B, Thomas ED, Nathan DG, et al: Severe aplastic anemia: A prospective study of the effect of early marrow transplantation on acute mortality. Blood 1976;48:63–70.

8 Najean Y, Pecking A: Prognostic factors in acquired aplastic anemia. A study of 352 cases. Am J Med 1979;67:564–571.
9 Mir MA, Geary CG: Aplastic anemia: An analysis of 174 patients. Postgrad Med J 1980;56: 322–326.
10 Li FP, Alter BP, Nathan DG: The mortality of acquired aplastic anemia in children. Blood 1972;40:153–162.
11 Weiss G: Verlauf und Prognose der erworbenen Panmyelopathie; doct thesis, Ulm, 1980.
12 Schrezenmeier H, Marin P, Raghavachar A, et al: Relapse of aplastic anemia after immunosuppressive treatment: A report from the European Bone Marrow Transplantation Group SAA Working Party. Br J Haematol 1993;85: 371–377.
13 Camitta B, O'Reilly RJ, Sensenbrenner L, et al: Antithoracic duct lymphocyte globulin therapy of severe aplastic anemia. Blood 1983;62:883–888.
14 Champlin R, Ho W, Gale RP: Antithymocyte globulin treatment in patients with aplastic anemia: A prospective randomized trial. N Engl J Med 1983;308:113–118.
15 Frickhofen N, Kaltwasser JP, Schrezenmeier H, et al: Treatment of aplastic anemia with antilymphocyte globulin and methylprednisolone with or without cyclosporine. N Engl J Med 1991;324:1297–1304.
16 Lewis SM: Course and prognosis in aplastic anemia. Br Med J 1965;i:1027–1031.
17 Te Velde J, Haak HL: Histology of bone marrow failure, a follow-up study in aplastic anaemia. Hämatol Bluttransfus 1979;24:15–25.
18 Lynch RE, Williams DM, Reading JC, et al: The prognosis in aplastic anemia. Blood 1975; 45:517–528.
19 Frisch B, Lewis SM: The bone marrow in aplastic anaemia: Diagnostic and prognostic features. J Clin Pathol 1974;27:231–241.
20 Camitta BM, Rappeport JM, Parkman R, Nathan DG: Selection of patients for bone marrow transplantation in severe aplastic anemia. Blood 1975;45:355–363.
21 Alter BP, Potter NU, Li FP: Classification and aetiology of the aplastic anemias. Clin Haematol 1978;7:431-465.
22 Lohrmann HP, Niethammer D, Kern P, et al: Identification of high-risk patients with aplastic anaemia in selection for allogeneic bone-marrow transplantation. Lancet 1976;ii:647–650.
23 Heimpel H: Epidemiology and etiology of aplastic anemia; in Bacigalupo A, Schrezenmeier H (eds): Aplastic Anemia: Pathophysiology and Therapy. Cambridge, Cambridge University Press, 1999, pp 97–116.
24 Camitta BM, Nathan DG, Forman EN, et al: Posthepatitic severe aplastic anemia – an indication for early bone marrow transplantation. Blood 1974;43:473–483.
25 Brown KE, Tisdale J, Barrett AJ, et al: Hepatitis-associated aplastic anemia. N Engl J Med 1997;336:1059-1064.
26 Keisu M, Heit W, Lambertenghi Deliliers G, et al: Transient pancytopenia. A report from the International Agranulocytosis and Aplastic Study. Blut 1990;61:240–244.
27 Heimpel H, Kubanek B: Pathophysiology of aplastic anaemia. Br J Haematol 1975;31 (suppl):57–68.
28 Camitta BM, Storb R, Thomas ED: Aplastic anemia. II. Pathogenesis, diagnosis, treatment, and prognosis. N Engl J Med 1982;306:712–718.
29 Tichelli A, Gratwohl A, Nissen C, et al: Spätkomplikationen bei Patienten mit aplastischer Anämie. Schweiz Med Wochenschr 1988;118: 1528–1532.
30 Tichelli A, Gratwohl A, Nissen C, et al: Morphology in patients with severe aplastic anemia treated with antilymphocyte globulin. Blood 1992;80:337–345.
31 Tichelli A, Gratwohl A, Nissen C, et al: Late clonal complications in severe aplastic anemia. Leuk Lymphoma 1994;12:167–175.
32 De Planque MM, Kluin-Nelemans HC, van Krieken HJ, et al: Evolution of acquired severe aplastic anaemia to myelodysplasia and subsequent leukaemia in adults. Br J Haematol 1988;70:55–62.
33 Frickhofen N, Kaltwasser JP, Heimpel H, et al: 10-year results of a German phase III trial evaluation treatment of aplastic anemia with antithymocyte globulin with and without cyclosporin A (abstract), in press.
34 Gordon-Smith E: Treatment of aplastic anemia. I. Conservative management; in Geary CG (ed): Aplastic Anemia. London, Baillière Tindall, 1979, pp 108–130.
35 The International Agranulocytosis and Aplastic Anemia Study: Incidence of aplastic anemia: The relevance of diagnostic criteria. Blood 1987;70:1718–1821.
36 Heimpel H: Stimulation of hemopoiesis in aplastic anemia by hormones and other agents; in Heimpel H, Gordon-Smith EC, Heit W, et al (eds): Aplastic Anemia – Pathophysiology and Approaches to Therapy. Berlin, Springer, 1979, pp 129–137.
37 Shahidi NT, Diamond LK: Testosteron-induced remission in aplastic anemia of both acquired and congenital type. N Engl J Med 1961;266:953.
38 Bock EL, Fülle HH, Heimpel H, et al: Die Wirkung von Mesterolone bei Panmyelopathien und renaler Anämie. Med Klin 1976;71:539–547.
39 Branda RF, Amsden TW, Jacob HS: Randomized study of nandrolone therapy for anemias due to bone marrow failure. Arch Intern Med 1977;137:65–69.
40 Camitta BM, Thomas ED: Severe aplastic anaemia: A prospective study of the effect of androgens or transplantation on haematological recovery and survival. Clin Haematol 1978; 7:587–595.
41 Champlin RE, Ho WG, Feig SA, et al: Do androgens enhance the response to antithymocyte globulin in patients with aplastic anemia? A prospective randomized trial. Blood 1985; 66:184–188.
42 Bacigalupo A, Chaple M, Hows J, et al: Treatment of aplastic anaemia (AA) with antilymphocyte globulin (ALG) and methylprednisolone (MPred) with or without androgens: A randomized trial from the EBMT SAA working party. Br J Haematol 1993;83:145–151.
43 Kaltwasser JP, Dix U, Schalk KP, et al: Effect of androgens on the response to antithymocyte globulin in patients with aplastic anaemia. Eur J Haematol 1988;40:111–118.
44 Najean Y, Pecking A: Androgen therapy in aplastic anemia: short- and long-term results of a cooperative trial in 252 cases; in Najean Y (ed): Medullary Aplasia. New York, Masson, 1980, pp 205–211.
45 Tso SC, Chan TK, Todd D: Aplastic anaemia: A study of prognosis and the effect of androgen therapy. Q J Med 1977;46:513–529.
46 Azen EA, Shahidi NT: Androgen dependency in acquired aplastic anemia. Am J Med 1977; 63:320–324.
47 Pizzuto J, Conte G, Sinco A, et al: Use of androgens in acquired aplastic anaemia. Relation of response to aetiology and severity. Acta Haematol 1980;64:18–24.
48 Olmer J, Carcassonne Y: La splénectomie dans les pancytopénies idiopathiques. Presse Méd 1960;68:857–860.
49 Heaton LD, Crosby WH, Cohen A: Splenectomy in the treatment of hypoplasia of the bone marrow. Ann Surg 1957;146:637.
50 Dreyfus B: A propos de 81 observations de pancytopénies idiopathiques chroniques sans splénomegalie. Rev franc Hématol 1959;14:62.
51 Heimpel H: Die Panmyelopathie und andere Formen der Pancytopenie; in Schwiegk H (ed): Handbuch der Inneren Medizin. Heidelberg, Springer, 1974, pp 83–134.
52 Speck B, Tichelli A, Widmer E, et al: Splenectomy as an adjuvant measure in the treatment of severe aplastic anaemia. Br J Haematol 1996; 92:818–824.
53 Ascensao JL, Pahwa R, Kagan W, et al: Aplastic anaemia: Evidence for an immunological mechanism. Lancet 1976;i:669–671.
54 Heimpel H, Dietrich M, Erdmann H: Azathioprinbehandlung einer kindlichen Panmyelopathie mit schwerer amegakaryozytärer Thrombozytopenie. Verh Dtsch Ges Inn Med 1968; 74:631.

Acta Hæmatologica

Acta Haematol 2000;103:16–18

# What Is the Definition of Cure for Aplastic Anemia?

Bruce M. Camitta

Midwest Children's Cancer Center, Department of Pediatrics, Medical College of Wisconsin and the Children's Hospital of Wisconsin, Milwaukee, Wisc., USA

**Key Word**
Aplastic anemia · Cure · Definition

**Abstract**
Treatment with immune suppression and bone marrow transplantation has improved the response rates and survival of patients with aplastic anemia. Measurement of response requires that common endpoints be recorded at specific times. There has been no agreement on such parameters for patients with aplastic anemia. In this paper issues related to measurement of response are reviewed and criteria for response are proposed. Adoption of uniform criteria would facilitate comparisons of treatment efficacy.



The past three decades have witnessed significant improvements in both survival and hematologic responses of patients with aplastic anemia. These reflect an increased understanding of the pathogenesis of marrow aplasia, better supportive care (transfusions, antibiotics), and more effective treatment (immune suppression, bone marrow transplantation). However, after immune suppression, hematologic recovery is frequently incomplete, relapses are common, and patients are at increased risk for the development of other marrow diseases, such as paroxysmal nocturnal hemoglobinuria (PNH), myelodysplasia (MDS) and acute nonlymphocytic leukemia (ANLL). Patients treated with bone marrow transplantation also may have suboptimal hematopoietic recovery and are at increased risks for complications of the preparatory regimen, graft-versus-host disease and delayed immune reconstitution.

Measurement of response to treatment requires that particular parameters (endpoints) be recorded at specified periods of time. Unfortunately, for patients with aplastic anemia, investigators have used multiple endpoints to define response. In this paper, issues related to the measurement of response of patients with aplastic anemia are explored. Criteria for definitions of response are proposed. Adoption of such uniform criteria would facilitate evaluations of treatment efficacy and comparisons of results between trials in the same way as the use of a common definition of disease severity [1].

## Problems with Defining Cure

*Blood and Marrow Counts.* At diagnosis, patients with aplastic anemia have decreased numbers of hematopoietic stem cells, a hypocellular bone marrow and peripheral blood cytopenias. Residual stem cells function poorly. Following treatment, peripheral recovery is often incomplete (especially for patients treated with immune suppression). Less well appreciated are the persistent deficits in both numbers and functioning of hematopoietic stem cells [2, 3]. This is true for patients treated with either immune suppression or bone marrow transplantation. Thus, if full hematopoietic recovery is used as the measure of response, most patients with aplastic anemia are never cured.

KARGER
Fax +41 61 306 12 34
E-Mail karger@karger.ch
www.karger.com

© 2000 S. Karger AG, Basel
0001–5792/00/1031–0016$17.50/0

Accessible online at:
www.karger.com/journals/aha

Bruce Camitta, MD
Midwest Children's Cancer Center, MACC Fund Research Center
8701 Watertown Plank Rd
Milwaukee, WI 53226 (USA)
Tel. +1 414 456 4106, Fax +1 414 456 6543, E-Mail bcamitta@mcw.edu

A related issue is the use of varied complete blood count (CBC) criteria for declaring response. This is especially perplexing when a patient is declared to have had a complete response. It would seem logical to use published normal values as the appropriate criteria for complete response. Use of lesser values enhances study statistics at the expense of blurring reality.

*Time to Response.* Most responses to immune suppression begin within 4 months of initial treatment [1, 4, 5]. Responses that begin more than 6–8 months after treatment are more likely to be due to prolonged survival than to therapy per se. Therefore, in most instances, a lack of response at 8 months should be coded as a failure of that therapy.

*Duration of Response.* How long must hematologic improvement persist before a patient is deemed to have responded? Clearly, a single CBC is inadequate. However, different studies have required that blood counts remain above specified levels for 1 week to 2 months before response status is confirmed. Since transient responses are of little value to the patient, it would seem prudent to require that improvement last for at least 1 month before a patient is declared to have responded.

*Continued Cytokine Support.* Use of G-CSF, GM-CSF or other cytokines increases the number of neutrophils in most patients with aplastic anemia [4]. However, upon withdrawal of cytokine treatment, neutrophil counts usually fall to lower levels. It would appear logical to require that cytokine support has been discontinued for at least 2 weeks before the initial CBC that uses neutrophil levels to declare response. This requirement would apply equally to patients who are treated with cytokines alone or in combination with immune suppressive therapy. Alternatively, reports should clearly specify what percent of responding patients are still receiving one or more cytokines.

*Relapse.* Approximately 25–50% of patients who respond to immune suppression eventually have a hematologic relapse [6–8]. Recurrence of aplastic anemia is rare after bone marrow transplantation. Although secondary treatments may salvage many patients who relapse [8], success of salvage treatment should not be credited to the initial therapy.

*Clonal Evolution.* Approximately 25–60% of patients treated with immune suppression develop other marrow diseases: PNH, MDS or ANLL [6, 7, 9]. This may reflect emergence of previously undetected abnormal clones that were present at initial diagnosis of aplastic anemia. Alternatively, damaged hematopoietic stem cells may be more susceptible to accumulation of additional genetic insults. The risks of developing MDS or ANLL appear to be higher in older patients and in patients who have received more than one course of immune suppression [9]. Development of MDS or ANLL should be treated as signaling the end of hematologic response.

*Other Complications.* Clear delineation of acute and chronic toxicities is important for the comparison of responses to treatments. Fever, hemolysis, hypotension and serum sickness are common acute problems in patients treated with antilymphocyte globulin. Graft versus host disease (acute and chronic) is a risk of bone marrow transplantation regardless of conditioning regimen. For patients prepared for transplantation with irradiation, endocrine abnormalities, fertility problems, cataracts, lung disease, renal abnormalities, venocclusive disease and solid tumors are frequent problems [9, 10]. Although each of these problems may affect long-term survival, follow-up in most reports is more short term.

*Event-Free Survival versus Survival.* Event-free survival is the measure of choice for assessing the response to a specific treatment. As applied to patients with aplastic anemia, failure of event-free survival occurs after initial failure to respond, relapse, development of MDS or ANLL, or death from any cause. Survival, on the other hand, reflects not only the primary treatment but also the effects of any salvage treatments. However, reporting survival may be of value for comparing whether one sequence of treatments is better than another (for example, immune suppression followed by marrow transplantation or the reverse sequence). Whatever endpoint is selected, actuarial methods which account for unequal follow-up are mandatory. Also note that in an intervention trial where divergence between treatments occurs after a given point, randomization should occur at the point of divergence and the primary endpoint should be event-free (or disease-free) survival after divergence. This minimizes the number of patients required to meet the study objectives.

**Table 1.** General guidelines for evaluating responses to treatment of aplastic anemia

| | |
|---|---|
| 1 | Use established normal values for CBC results |
| 2 | Responses should be confirmed by 2 or more CBCs at least 4 weeks apart |
| 3 | Responses ideally should be measured in patients who are not receiving colony-stimulating factors. If one or more of these factors are still being given, this should be specified |
| 4 | Event-free survival or disease-free survival are preferable to survival for evaluating response to specific therapy. Failure to respond, death from any cause, relapse and clonal evolution (MDS, ANLL) all signal the end of event-free survival. Only death, relapse and cloncal evolution affect disease-free survival |

**Table 2.** Response criteria for treatment of aplastic anemia

| | | | | |
|---|---|---|---|---|
| *Severe aplastic anemia* | | | | |
| None | still severe | | | |
| Partial | transfusion independent | | | |
| | no longer meeting criteria for severe disease | | | |
| Complete | hemoglobin normal for age | | | |
| | PMN $>1,500/\mu l$ | | | |
| | platelets $>150,000/\mu l$ | | | |
| *Mild aplastic anemia* | | | | |
| None | worse or not meeting criteria below | | | |
| Partial | transfusion independence (if previously required) | | | |
| | *or* doubling or normalization of at least one cell line | | | |
| | *or* increase above baseline | hemoglobin | 3 g/dl | (if initially $<6$) |
| | | PMN | $500/\mu l$ | (if initially $<500$) |
| | | platelets | $20,000/\mu l$ | (if initially $<20,000$) |
| Complete | same criteria as for severe disease | | | |

## Recommendations

Uniform reporting of responses to treatment of aplastic anemia is necessary if we are to optimize the information obtained from individual trials. Table 1 lists general guidelines. In table 2, definitions of response are suggested. These definitions were developed at an international conference in Santa Margherita Ligure in 1998. The criteria for patients with severe aplastic anemia are relatively straightforward. The criteria for patients with milder disease may require eventual reworking. However, it is suggested that the definitions in table 2 be given an initial trial.

Using these guidelines, the ideal way to present response data includes: (a) a statement or table of the maximum responses attained; (b) an actuarial graph of the time required to achieve partial and complete responses; (c) data indicating the numbers of patients with complete and partial responses who relapse or develop clonal disease (and the timing of these events); (d) an actuarial graph of event-free survival (which begins at 100%) or disease-free survival (which begins at 100% – nonresponding %). In either graph, events include relapse, death and clonal evolution; (e) an accounting of the results of secondary treatments given separately for patients with each type of failure (nonresponse, relapse and clonal evolution), and (f) an actuarial graph of survival.

The ability to compare outcomes of different studies or treatments is critical for the advancement of knowledge. At the present time, few studies (including the author's) of the treatment of aplastic anemia comply with most of the above recommendations. It is incumbent on investigators in this field to justify our patients' trust by maximizing the information obtained from the study of their disease.

## References


1 Camitta BM, Thomas ED, Nathan DG, et al: A prospective study of androgens and bone marrow transplantation for treatment of severe aplastic anemia. Blood 1976;53:504–514.

2 Maciejewski JP, Selleri C, Sato T, Anderson S, Young NS: A severe and consistent deficit in marrow and circulating primitive hematopoietic stem cells (long-term culture-initiating cells) in acquired aplastic anemia. Blood 1996;88:1983–1991.

3 Schrezenmeier H, Jenal M, Herrmann F, Heimpel H, Raghavachar A: Quantitative analysis of cobblestone area-forming cells in bone marrow of patients with aplastic anemia by limiting dilution assay. Blood 1996;88:4474–4480.

4 Camitta B, O'Reilly R, Sensenbrenner L, et al: Antithoracic duct lymphocyte globulin therapy of severe aplastic anemia. Blood 1983;62:883–888.

5 Bacigalupo A, Broccia G, Corda G, et al: Antilymphocyte globulin, cyclosporine, and granulocyte colony-stimulating factor in patients with acquired severe aplastic anemia (SAA): A pilot study of the EBMT SAA working party. Blood 1995;85:1348–1353.

6 Tichelli A, Gratwohl A, Wursch A, et al: Late haematological complications in severe aplastic anaemia. Br J Haematol 1988;69:413–418.

7 de Planque NNM, Bacigalupo A, Wursch A, et al: Long-term follow-up of severe aplastic anaemia patients treated with antithymocyte globulin. Br J Haematol 1989;73:121–126.

8 Rosenfeld SJ, Young NS: Aplastic anemia treated by immunosuppression is a chronic relapsing illness, but prognosis is unaffected by relapse. Blood 1997;90(suppl 1):435a.

9 Socie G, Amar MH, Bacigalupo A, et al: Malignancies occurring after treatment of aplastic anemia: A survey conducted by the Severe Aplastic Anemia working party of the European Group for Bone Marrow Transplantation. N Engl J Med 1993;329:1152–1161.

10 Deeg HJ, Leisenring W, Storb R, et al: Long-term outcome after marrow transplantation for severe aplastic anemia. Blood 1998;91:3637–3645.

Acta Hæmatologica

Acta Haematol 2000;103:19–25

# Current Results of Bone Marrow Transplantation in Patients with Acquired Severe Aplastic Anemia

## Report of the European Group for Blood and Marrow Transplantation

A. Bacigalupo R. Oneto B. Bruno G. Socié J. Passweg A. Locasciulli M.T. Van Lint A. Tichelli S. McCann J. Marsh P. Ljungman J. Hows P. Marin H. Schrezenmeier

on behalf of the Working Party on Severe Aplastic Anemia of the European Group for Blood and Marrow Transplantation, and the Medical Statistical Department, University of Leiden, The Netherlands

**Key Words**

Aplastic anemia · Bone marrow transplantation · GvHD · Rejection · Radiotherapy

**Abstract**

We have analyzed 2,002 patients grafted in Europe between 1976 and 1998 from an identical twin (n = 34), from an HLA-identical sibling (n = 1,699) or from an alternative donor (n = 269), which included unrelated and family mismatched donors. The proportions of patients surviving in these three groups are, respectively, 91, 66 and 37%: major causes of failure were acute graft-versus host disease (GvHD) (11%), infection (12%), pneumonitis (4%), rejection (4%). In multivariate Cox analysis, factors predicting outcome were patient's age ($p < 0.0001$), donor type ($p < 0.0001$), interval between diagnosis and bone marrow transplantation (BMT) ($p < 0.0005$), year of BMT ($p = 0.0005$) and female donor for a male recipient ($p = 0.02$). Patients were then divided in two groups according to the year of BMT: up to or after 1990. The overall death rate dropped from 43 to 24% ($p < 0.00001$). Improvements were seen mostly for grafts from identical siblings (from 54 to 75%, $p < 0.0001$), and less so for alternative-donor grafts (from 28 to 35%; $p = 0.07$). Major changes have occurred in the BMT protocol: decreasing use of radiotherapy in the conditioning regimen (from 35 to 24%; $p < 0.0001$) and increasing use of cyclosporin (with or without methotrexate) for GvHD prophylaxis (from 70 to 98%; $p < 0.0001$). In conclusion, the outcome of allogeneic BMT for patients with severe aplastic anemia has considerably improved over the past two decades: young patients, grafted early after diagnosis from an identical sibling, have currently an over 80% chance of long-term survival. Transplants from twins are very successful as well. The risk of complications with alternative donor transplants is still high.



## Introduction

Bone marrow transplantation (BMT) for severe aplastic anemia (SAA) was introduced in the early seventies and is still considered as the first-line therapy for young patients. The original conditioning regimen described by Santos and Owens [1] consisted of cyclophosphamide, 200 mg/kg, and was then used by Storb et al [2–5] in the first systematic series of patients. BMT has since then been the treatment of choice for patients with aplastic

KARGER

Fax + 41 61 306 12 34
E-Mail karger@karger.ch
www.karger.com


0001–5792/00/1031–0019$17.50/0

Accessible online at:
www.karger.com/journals/aha

A. Bacigalupo
Second Department of Haematology
Ospedale San Martino, Servizio Radioterapia IST
I–16132 Genoa (Italy)
Tel. +39 010 355 469, Fax +39 010 355 583, E-Mail apbacigalupo@smartino.ge.it

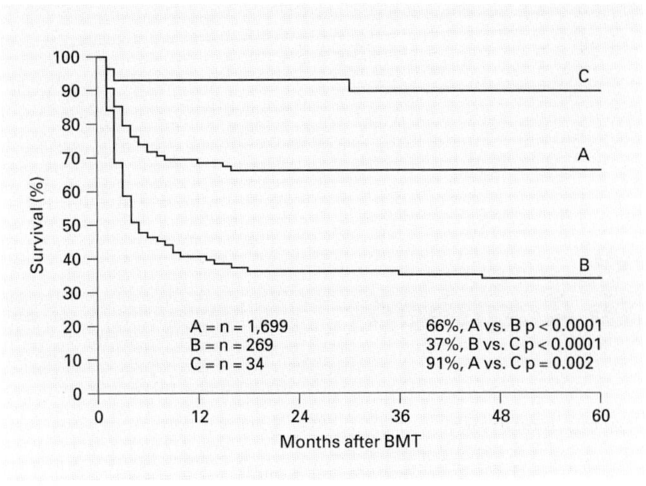


**Fig. 1.** Actuarial survival at 5 years among patients undergoing a BMT from HLA-identical siblings (A), alternative donors (B) or syngeneic twin (C).

**Table 1.** Patients' characteristics

| | |
|---|---|
| Number | 2,002 |
| Age, years | |
| Median | 18 |
| Range | 1–69 |
| Gender | |
| Males | 1,214 |
| Females | 750 |
| Unknown | 38 |
| Etiology | |
| Idiopathic | 1,370 |
| Hepatitis | 160 |
| Drug induced | 84 |
| Other | 388 |
| BMT | |
| Until 1990 | 1,091 |
| After 1990 | 911 |
| Severity of neutropenia | |
| 0.2 × $10^9$/l | 57% |
| 0.2–0.5 × $10^9$/l | 21% |
| 0.5 × $10^9$/l | 20% |
| Neutrophil count at BMT | |
| Median, × $10^9$/l | 0.2 |
| Range, × $10^9$/l | 0–4.9 |
| Interval between diagnosis and BMT | |
| Median, days | 96 |
| Range, days | 1–11,198 |

anemia and a suitable donor in the family [1–10, 16–18]. In the present study, we are reporting patients with acquired aplastic anemia from the Registry of the Working Party on SAA of the European Group for Blood and Marrow Transplantation (WPSAA EBMT). Patients with Fanconi's anemia, Diamond Blakfan syndrome and paroxysmal nocturnal hemoglobinuria were excluded from this analysis.

## Patients and Methods

2002 patients received a BMT between 1971 and 1998 (median year of BMT: 1991). The clinical characteristics of these patients are outlined in table 1. The median age was, respectively, 19, 15, 22 years for patients grafted from an HLA-identical sibling (n = 1,699), an alternative donor (n = 269) or a twin (n = 31), with a significant difference between the first two (p = 0.0004). The median interval between diagnosis and BMT was 97, 303 and 84 days, respectively ($p < 0.001$).

Two hundred and sixty-five (13%) patients had received immunosuppressive therapy before BMT: this number has dropped from 18% before 1985 to 17% <1990, to 10% <1995 to 4% in 1995+.

## Results

### *Survival*

The proportion of patients surviving is 66, 37 and 91% for patients grafted from an HLA-identical sibling, an alternative donor, or an identical twin (fig. 1). Median follow-up for surviving patients in these three groups is, respectively, 1,430 days (5–8,843), 820 days (18–6,284), 2,643 days (36–6,565). Median follow-up for patients who died after BMT in these three groups is, respectively, 79 days (1–5,535), 62 days (1–2,759), 32 days (8–874).

### *Causes of Failure*

The major causes of failure were acute graft-versus-host disease (GvHD) (11%), infection (12%), pneumonitis (4%), rejection (4%). Mortality due to GvHD, infection, rejection and pneumonitis was significantly greater among patients who received a graft from an alternative donor. Mortality has dropped from 43% up to 1990 to 24% after 1990 ($p < 0.00001$), with a major decrease for GvHD-related deaths (14 to 5%) and less so for pneumonitis (5 to 2.5%), infection (14 to 9%) and rejection (4.7 to 2.4%).

### *Graft Failure and Rejection*

Rejection correlates with donor type: patients receiving grafts from alternative donors (family mismatched

**Table 2.** Patients undergoing BMT in Europe 1976–1998 (EBMT data 1998)

| Origin of graft | n | Median age years | Interval $D_x$–$T_x$, days | Graft failure, % | GvHD % | Surviving n | Surviving % | >1 BMT % |
|---|---|---|---|---|---|---|---|---|
| Identical twin | 34 | 22 | 84 | 10 | 0 | 31 | 91 | 38 |
| HLA-identical sibling | 1,699 | 19 | 97 | 12 | 13 | 1,116 | 66 | 8 |
| Alternative donor | 269 | 15 | 303 | 26 | 28 | 101 | 37 | 12 |

$D_x$–$T_x$ = Median interval between diagnosis and treatment in days; GvHD = acute GvHD grade III.

and unrelated ) had a significantly higher rate of graft failure/rejection when compared to HLA-identical sibling BMT, i.e. 26 vs. 12% (p < 0.00001); they also had a significantly greater risk of needing a second BMT (p < 0.0001) (table 2). The risk was highest for those receiving grafts from twins, among whom 38% received more than 1 graft, due to the fact that some of them had not been conditioned for the first graft.

When we looked only at patients receiving grafts from HLA-identical siblings, there was a decrease in graft failure with time, but this decrease was not as dramatic as expected: 18% before 1980, 12% in 1980–1990 and 11% in 1991–1998 (p = 0.12). In the last 10 years, a persisting small proportion of patients has failed to engraft or reject, especially if conditioned with cyclophosphamide alone (9%); this proportion may have been reduced by the addition of antilymphocyte globulin (ALG) (0% rejections).

*Effect of Age*

The effect of age in transplants from HLA-identical siblings is clear, with a decrease in survival for each decade. Survival at age <10 years, <20, <30, <40, and >40 is, respectively, 68, 64, 61, 54, 54 and 43%. In the years 1976–1989, the actuarial survival of patients aged <16, 17–40, >40 was, respectively, 60, 53 and 27% (p < 0.0001). In the years 1990–1998, it is 77, 68 and 54% (p < 0.001). The effect has remained although the outcome is superior in all age groups.

*Role of Radiotherapy in the Conditioning Regimen*

Among the 1,699 patients who had received grafts from HLA-identical siblings, 531 had radiotherapy as part of their conditioning regimen, in the form of total body irradiation or thoraco-abdominal irradiation [5] or total lymphoid irradiation. The actuarial 5-year survival of patients given irradiation is 62% compared to 64% for patients prepared without irradiation (p = 0.1). The crude incidence of chronic GvHD in patients receiving irradiation is 34 vs. 23% (p < 0.0001) and the crude rate of malignant disease is 4 vs. 1% (p = 0.001). Therefore there is no survival advantage for patients receiving irradiation, and there is a higher incidence of late complications such as chronic GvHD and malignant disease.

The crude survival of 551 patients receiving cyclophosphamide alone as conditioning agent and cyclosporin with or without methotrexate for GvHD prophylaxis is 69%; the addition of ALG in the conditioning regimen was recorded in 28 patients; their survival is 87% (confirming the excellent results reported by Storb et al. [5]).

*Acute GvHD*

Acute GvHD was recorded as grades 0–I , II and III–IV in 75, 11 and 13% of patients, respectively. Grade III–IV acute GvHD was scored in 20% before 1990 and in 6% of patients from 1990 onward (p < 0.00001). This is mainly, but not exclusively, due to changes in GvHD prophylaxis regimens: the incidence of severe (grade III–IV) acute GvHD was 26% for methotrexate prophylaxis, 11% for cyclosporin, and 9% for cyclosporin + methotrexate (p < 0.00001). The actuarial survival is profoundly influenced by acute GvHD: for grades 0–I, II, and III–IV, the actuarial 5-year survival is 60, 55 and 32% in 1976–1989 (p < 0.00001) and 77, 60 and 33% in 1990–1998 (p < 0.0001). It is interesting to note that the improved survival is seen exclusively among patients with GvHD grade 0–I, whereas patients with GvHD grades II and III–IV have not improved.

*Chronic GvHD*

Chronic GvHD in patients surviving for 100 days was recorded as absent in 77%, limited in 13% and extensive in 10%. As with acute GvHD, extensive chronic GvHD has also decreased from 15% before 1990 to 5% in 1990–1998 (p < 0.00001). The overall actuarial survival at

5 years for patients with no, limited or extensive chronic GvHD is 89, 84 and 55%. Survival beyond day 100 has not changed before or after 1990, suggesting that (a) improved outcome is due to reduction in early deaths and (b) patients with extensive chronic GvHD are still at risk of dying. In conclusion, GvHD has a significant impact on survival. Because the risk of developing severe acute or chronic GvHD is significantly lower at present, survival of patients with SAA after BMT from an HLA-identical sibling has improved. However, our ability to treat GvHD has not improved over the years.

*Effect of Year of BMT*

The overall death rate has dropped from 43% before 1990 to 24% in the period 1990–1998 ($p < 0.00001$). The improvement of outcome has been more significant for identical-sibling transplants (from 54 to 75%, $p < 0.0001$), and less so for alternative donor grafts (from 28 to 35%, $p = 0.07$).

## Conclusions

The present report confirms that outcome after BMT for aplastic anaemia has significantly improved over the past two decades: this is mostly due to a reduction in early mortality, up to 100 days after BMT. In the two time periods analyzed (up to 1990 and after 1990), there has been a significant reduction in the number of patients with severe (grade III–IV) GvHD, and this has also resulted in less extensive chronic GvHD. If we look at patients stratified for the severity of acute GvHD, improvement is seen only in patients with grade 0–II and not III–IV, and the same is true for chronic GvHD. Therefore, we have improved our ability to prevent severe GvHD, both in its acute and chronic form, and we now see less patients with extensive disease; however, if severe GvHD develops, our ability to treat remains low.

There has been a reduction in rejection, although our understanding of graft failure is more accurate today: we now have information on mixed chimerism after BMT and we know that a considerable proportion of patients exhibit some degree of autologous reconstitution after cyclophosphamide alone, which can be transient, persistent or progressive, leading to rejection [12, 13]. A major reduction in graft failure occurred at the time when cyclosporin was introduced, in the early eighties.

Irradiation has been increasingly used until the early nineties, when one third of the patients were prepared with some form of irradiation. The use of radiotherapy has been declining since, due to reports on secondary malignancies [19, 20], although at present still approximately 25% of patients receiving grafts from HLA-identical siblings are prepared with conditioning regimens that include irradiation, and we believe this should be firmly discouraged. Irradiation produces more chronic GvHD, more pneumonitis and does not improve survival [9, 19, 20].

The vast majority of transplants in the Registry are from HLA-identical sibling donors. It is important that young patients are grafted early in the course of the disease, with no irradiation in the conditioning regimen and with cyclosporin/methotrexate for GvHD prophylaxis. Transplants from alternative donors still have a poor prognosis: results have not improved significantly, and 5-year survival in the order of 40% can be expected: causes of failure are graft rejection and GvHD. New conditioning regimens, either with reduced doses of irradiation or with fludarabine are being explored.

## Acknowledgments

This work was supported by BIOMED EEC grant No. 951031 to H.S. and a grant from Associazione Italiana contro il Cancro, Milano, to A.B, and Associazione Ricerca Trapianto Midollo Osseo, Genova. We are grateful to all European centers who have contributed their data.

## Appendix: Centers Participating in the Current Study

| | | |
|---|---|---|
| 201 | Hôpital Necker | Paris |
| 202 | University Hospital | Basel |
| 203 | University Hospital | Leiden |
| 204 | Universität Ulm | Ulm |
| 205 | Hammersmith Hospital | London |
| 206 | Rigshospitalet | Copenhagen |
| 207 | Hôpital St. Louis | Paris |
| 208 | University Hospital | Zürich |
| 209 | Hematology, University Hospital | Leuven |
| 210 | Charing Cross-Westminster, Medical School | London |
| 212 | University Hospital | Huddinge |
| 213 | Hôpital Saint Antoine | Paris |
| 214 | Hospital Clinic | Barcelona |
| 215 | Institut Jules Bordet | Brussels |
| 216 | Royal Free Hospital | London |
| 217 | Ospedale San Martino | Genova |
| 218 | Marsden Hospital | Sutton |
| 219 | Children's Hospital | Helsinki |
| 222 | Hôtel Dieu | Paris |
| 223 | Medizinische Universitätsklinik | Tübingen |
| 224 | University College, London Hospital | London |
| 225 | Turku University | Turku |
| 226 | Servicio Ematologia, Medicina II | Cremona |
| 227 | BMT Unit, University Hospital | Vienna |
| 228 | Royal Infirmary | Edinburgh |
| 230 | Institut Paoli I. Calmettes | Marseille |
| 231 | Clinica Medica Università | Torino |
| 232 | Università degli Studi 'La Sapienza' | Roma |
| 233 | Hôpital Jean Minjoz | Besançon |
| 234 | Cliniques Universitaires St. Luc | Brussels |
| 235 | The National Hospital | Oslo |
| 236 | Hospital de la Princesa | Madrid |
| 237 | University Hospital St Radboud | Nijmegen |
| 238 | Hospital Reina Sofia | Cordoba |
| 239 | University Hospital | Utrecht |
| 240 | Hospital San Orsola | Bologna |
| 242 | Marquès de Valdecilla | Santander |
| 243 | Great Ormond Street Hospital | London |
| 244 | Glasgow Royal Infirmary | Glasgow |
| 246 | Dr. Daniel den Hoed Cancer Center | Rotterdam |
| 247 | Academic Medical Centre | Amsterdam |
| 248 | Ospedale Civile | Pescara |
| 250 | Hôpital Nord | Saint-Etienne |
| 251 | Hôpital Caen | Caen |
| 252 | Hôpital Henri Mondor | Créteil |
| 253 | Hôtel Dieu | Nantes |
| 254 | St. James's University Hospital | Leeds |
| 255 | The Oxford Radcliffe Hospital | Oxford |
| 256 | BMT Unit, Department of Internal Medicine | Kiel |
| 257 | St. James Hospital Trinity College | Dublin |
| 258 | Hadassah University Hospital | Jerusalem |
| 259 | University Hospital | Essen |
| 260 | Hospital Santa Creu i Sant Pau | Barcelona |
| 261 | Hôpital Cantonal Universitaire | Geneva |
| 262 | Pitié-Salpêtrière | Paris |
| 264 | Hôpital La Miletrie | Poitiers |
| 265 | Istituto Scienze Mediche, Università Milano | Milano |
| 266 | University Hospital | Uppsala |
| 267 | Hôpital du Haut Leveque | Pessac |
| 270 | Hôpital A. Michallon | Grenoble |
| 271 | University Hospital | Innsbruck |
| 273 | Centre Jaen Perrin | Clermont-Ferrand |
| 274 | Istituto G. Gaslini | Genova |
| 276 | Royal Victoria Infirmary | Newcastle-upon-Tyne |
| 279 | Ospedale San Gerardo | Monza |
| 280 | Hôpital Cochin | Paris |
| 282 | Hospital Clinico Universitario | Valencia |
| 283 | University Hospital | Lund |
| 284 | Birmingham Heartlands Hospital | Birmingham |
| 285 | 2nd Clinica Pediatrica | Padova |
| 286 | Policlinico San Matteo | Pavia |
| 287 | S. Camillo Hospital | Roma |
| 288 | Ospedale Civile | Brescia |
| 289 | II. Medizinische Klinik, Städtisches Klinikum | Karlsruhe |
| 291 | Inst. Portugues Oncologia, BMT Unit | Porto |
| 292 | University Hospital Hacettepe | Ankara |
| 293 | Abteilung Innere Medizin, Virchow Klinikum | Berlin |
| 294 | Ospedale Niguarda Ca' Granda | Milano |
| 295 | Medical School Hannover | Hannover |
| 297 | Universität Frankfurt | Frankfurt |
| 300 | Inst. Portugues Oncologia | Lisboa |
| 301 | Hôpital d'Enfants de la Timone | Marseille |
| 304 | Ospedale di Careggi | Firenze |
| 305 | Ospedale Regina Margherita | Torino |
| 317 | HCI International Medical Centre | Clydebank |
| 332 | Istituto di Ematologia | Taranto |
| 336 | Klinikum und Poliklinikum Kinderheilkunde, Schwerpunkt: KMT | Berlin |
| 345 | Rambam Medical Center | Haifa |
| 349 | Département Hémato-Oncologie CHNDRF | Charleroi |
| 372 | Gata Military Medical Academy | Ankara |
| 386 | Bristol Hospital for Sick Children | Bristol |
| 390 | Heinrich Heine Universität | Düsseldorf |
| 392 | Ospedale V. Cervello – USL 60 | Palermo |
| 397 | King Faisal Specialist Hospital | Riyadh |
| 398 | University Hospital | Leiden |
| 501 | Royal Liverpool University Hospital | Liverpool |
| 504 | National Institute of Hematology and Immunology | Budapest |
| 512 | Department of Hematology, UCT Medical School | Cape Town |
| 513 | Klinikum Grosshadern | München |
| 515 | Helsinki University Central Hospital | Helsinki |
| 521 | Royal Manchester Children's Hospital | Pendlebury |
| 523 | Médecine Interne I, Hôpital Cimiez | Nice |
| 525 | Istituto per l'Infanzia Burlo Garofolo | Trieste |
| 527 | Hospital M. Infantil Vall d'Hebron | Barcelona |
| 528 | St. Anna Kinderspital | Wien |
| 529 | Pesaro Hospital | Pesaro |
| 535 | University Hospital | Tübingen |
| 538 | Dluski Hospital and Institute of Immunology and Experimental Therapy | Wroclaw |

➤

**Appendix** (continued)

| | | |
|---|---|---|
| 539 | St. George's Hospital Medical School | London |
| 557 | IRCCS Policlinico San Matteo | Pavia |
| 561 | The George Papanicolaou General Hospital | Exokhi |
| 566 | Addenbrooke's Hospital | Cambridge |
| 567 | Groupe Hospitalier Paul-Brousse | Villejuif |
| 576 | Hospital Regional de Malaga | Malaga |
| 581 | Wellington Hospital | Wellington |
| 582 | Military Medical Academy | Belgrade |
| 583 | R.G. Vall d'Hebron | Barcelona |
| 587 | Azienda Ospedaliera 'Bianchi-Melacrino-Morelli' | Reggio Calabria |
| 589 | Centre Hospitalier Universitaire | Clermont-Ferrand |
| 592 | Hämatologie und Onkologie | Idar-Oberstein |
| 593 | University Childrens Hospital | Graz |
| 594 | Elisabethinen-Hospital | Linz |
| 595 | Alfred Hospital | Melbourne |
| 598 | Hospital Nuestra Señora Aranzazu | San Sebastian |
| 599 | Postgraduate Medical School | Miskolc |
| 601 | Royal Infirmary | Manchester |
| 610 | University Hospital | Bratislava |
| 614 | Universitätskrankenhaus Eppendorf | Hamburg |
| 617 | Ibni Sina Hospital | Ankara |
| 622 | Evangelismos Hospital | Athens |
| 624 | Hôpital de Purpan | Toulouse |
| 630 | University Hospital VUB | Brussels |
| 631 | Hôpital Robert Debre | Paris |
| 633 | Shariati Hospital | Teheran |
| 640 | University Medical Center | Ljubljana |
| 641 | K. Marcinkowski University of Medical Science | Poznan |
| 642 | Hospital Covadonga | Oviedo |
| 644 | Children University Hospital | Brussels |
| 648 | Universiteit Antwerpen (UZA) | Antwerp-Edegem |
| 650 | Service des Maladies du Sang | Angers |
| 651 | Heinrich Heine Universität | Düsseldorf |
| 655 | Clinic of Hematology | Novi Sad |
| 656 | Institute of Hematology and Blood Transfusion | Praha |
| 658 | Ospedale Bergamo | Bergamo |
| 661 | Hôpital Sud (Hôpital Pontchaillou) | Rennes |
| 663 | Hospital Universitario La Fe | Valencia |
| 666 | Institut Gustave Roussy | Villejuif |
| 667 | Hôpital d'Enfants, CHU de Dijon | Dijon |
| 671 | Hôpital E. Herriot | Lyon |
| 672 | CHR-CHU-Hôpital de Hautepierre | Strasbourg |
| 675 | Hôpital Trousseau | Paris |
| 676 | Hôpital d'Enfants | Vandœuvre-lès-Nancy |
| 677 | SL.A.M. w. Katowicach | Katowice |
| 704 | University of Southampton | Southampton |
| 705 | Udine University Hospital | Udine |
| 710 | Royal Perth Hospital | Perth |
| 711 | The New Children's Hospital | Sydney |
| 713 | Leicester Royal Infirmary | Leicester |
| 714 | Marmara Universitesi Hastanesi | Istanbul |
| 715 | Sahlgrenska University Hospital | Goeteborg |
| 717 | Nottingham City Hospital | Nottingham |
| 718 | Charles University Hospital | Pilsen |
| 721 | Guy's Hospital, Department of Haematology | London |
| 722 | Hospital Son Dureta | Palma de Mallorca |
| 724 | Russian Institute of Hematology | St Petersburg |
| 726 | University of Liège | Liège |
| 727 | Hospital Clinico | Salamanca |
| 728 | Clinica Puerta de Hierro | Madrid |
| 729 | Charles University | Hradec Kr Lov |
| 730 | K. Marcinkowski University | Poznan |
| 734 | Hospital Infantil La Paz | Madrid |
| 735 | Hospital General Universitario | Murcia |
| 739 | St. László Hospital | Budapest |
| 741 | Università degli Studi di Brescia | Brescia |
| 742 | Antartida Hospital Privado | Buenos Aires |
| 744 | University Hospital Gent | Gent |
| 746 | University of Tartu | Tartu |
| 750 | University of Jena | Jena |
| 752 | 'Aghia Sophia' Children's Hospital | Athens |
| 755 | Schneider Children's Medical Center of Israel | Petach-Tikva |
| 756 | Università Tor Vergata | Roma |
| 759 | Institut Catala d'Oncologia | Barcelona |
| 760 | Istanbul Medical School | Instanbul |
| 761 | Cerrahpasa Medical School | Instanbul |
| 762 | Department of Pediatric Hematology/Oncology | Instanbul |
| 763 | King's Healthcare NHS Trust | London |
| 766 | University of Napoli | Napoli |
| 769 | Hospital Universitario 'Virgen del Rocio' | Sevilla |
| 772 | Cape Town Haematology Clinic | Wynberg |
| 773 | Alder Hay Children's Hospital | Liverpool |
| 774 | Our Lady's Hospital for Sick Children | Dublin |
| 776 | Llandough Hospital | Cardiff |
| 778 | The Roald Dahl | Sheffield |
| 781 | The Birmingham's Children's Hospital | Birmingham |
| 790 | University of Bologna | Bologna |
| 795 | University of Pisa | Pisa |
| 799 | Medical University of Gdansk | Gdansk |
| 801 | Hospital No. 9 | Minsk |
| 806 | Hôpital Debrousse | Lyon |
| 807 | Charité-Virchow Klinikum der Humboldt Universität | Berlin |
| 808 | Universitätsklinikum Dresden | Dresden |
| 809 | Department of Medicine III, University Erlangen | Erlangen |
| 810 | University of Freiburg | Freiburg |
| 812 | Ospedale Regionale Microcitemie | Cagliari |
| 816 | Military Medical Academie | Warszawa Szaserow |
| 818 | Riyadh Armed Forces Hospital | Riyadh |
| 819 | Hospital G.U. 'G. Maranon' | Madrid |
| 926 | Hôpital Lapeyronie | Montpellier |
| 932 | Hôpital Charles Nicolle | Rouen |
| 941 | Centre Rouen Becquerel | Rouen |
| 952 | Service Hématologie Pédiatrique | Toulouse |
| 953 | Hôpital de Hautepierre | Strasbourg |
| 988 | Hôpital Arnaud de Villeneuve | Montpellier |

## References

1 Santos GW, Owens AH Jr: Allogeneic marrow transplants in cyclophosphamide treated mice. Transplant Proc 1969;1:44–46.
2 Storb R, Thomas ED, Buckner CD, et al: Allogeneic marrow grafting for treatment of aplastic anaemia: A follow-up on long-term survivors. Blood 1976;48:817–841.
3 Storb R, Prentice RL, Thomas ED: Marrow transplantation for treatment of aplastic anemia. An analysis of factors associated with graft rejection. N Engl J Med 1977;296:61–65.
4 Storb R, Thomas ED for the Seattle Marrow Transplant Team: Marrow Transplantation for Treatment of Aplastic Anaemia. Clin Haematol 1978;7/3.
5 Storb R, Erzioni R, Anasetti C, Appelbaum FR, Buckner CD, Besinger W, Bryant E, Clift R, Deeg HJ, Doney K, Flowers M, Hansen J, Martin P, Pepe M, Sale G, Sanders J, Singer J, Sullivan KM, Thomas ED, Witerspoon RP: Cyclophosphamide combined with antithymocyte globulin in preparation for allogeneic marrow transplants in patients with aplastic anemia. Blood 1994;84:941–949.
6 Bacigalupo A, Hows J, Gluckman E, Nissen C, Marsh J, Van Lint MT, Congiu M, de Planque MM, Ernst P, McCann S, Ragavashar A, Frickhofen N, Wursch A, Marmont AM, Gordon-Smith EC, for the EBMT Working Party on Severe Aplastic Anaemia: Bone marrow transplantation (BMT) versus immunosuppression for the treatment of severe aplastic anaemia (SAA): A report of the EBMT SAA Working Party. Br J Haematol 1988;177:70.
7 Camitta BM, Thomas ED, Nathan DG, Gale RP, Kopecky KJ, Rapeport JM, Santos G, Gordon-Smith EC, Storb R: A prospective study of androgens and bone marrow transplantation for treatment of severe aplastic anemia. Blood 1979;53:504.
8 Champlin RE, Ho WG, Nimer SD, et al: Bone Marrow transplantation for severe aplastic anemia. Transplantation 1990;49:720–724.
9 Deeg HJ, Leisenring W, Storb R, Nims J, Flowers ME, Witherspoon RP, Sanders J, Sullivan KM: Long-term outcome after marrow transplantation for severe aplastic anemia. Blood 1998;91:3637–3645.
10 Doney K, Leisenring W, Storb R, Appelbaum FR: Primary treatment of acquired aplastic anemia: Outcomes with bone marrow transplantation and immunosuppressive therapy. Ann Intern Med 1997;126:107–115.
11 Gluckman E, Socié G, Devergie A, Bourdeau-Esperou H, Traineau R, Cosset JM: Bone marrow transplantation in 107 patients with severe aplastic anemia using cyclophosphamide and thoraco-abdominal irradiation for conditioning: Long-term follow-up. Blood 1993;78:2451–2455.
12 McCann SR, Lawler M: Mixed chimaerism: Detection and significance following BMT. Bone Marrow Transplant 1993;11:91–94.
13 McCann SR, Bacigalupo A, Gluckman E, Hinterberger W, Hows J, Ljungman P, Marin P, Nissen C, van't Veer Kerthof E, Raghavashar A, Socié G, Frickhofen N, Locasciulli A, Schrezenmeier H: Graft rejection and second bone marrow transplants for acquired aplastic anaemia: A report from the Aplastic Anaemia Working Party of the European Bone Marrow Transplant Group. Bone Marrow Transplant 1994;13:233–237.
14 McGlave PB, Haake R, Miller W, Kim T, Kersey J, Ramsay NKC: Therapy of severe aplastic anemia in young adults and children with allogeneic bone marrow transplantation. Blood 1987;70:1325–1330.
15 Passweg JR, Socié G, Hinterberger W, Bacigalupo A, Biggs JC, Camitta BM, Champlin RE, Gale RP, Gluckman E, Gordon-Smith EC, Hows JM, Klein JP, Nugent ML, Pasquini R, Rowlings PA, Speck B, Tichelli A, Zhang MJ, Horowitz MM, Bortin MM: Bone marrow transplantation for severe aplastic anemia: Has outcome improved? Blood 1997;90:858–864.
16 Speck B, Tichelli A, Gratwohl A, Nissen C: Treatment of severe aplastic anemia: A 12-year follow-up of patients after bone marrow transplantation or after therapy with antilymphocyte globulin; in Shahidi NT (ed): Aplastic Anemia and Other Bone Marrow Failure Syndromes. London, Springer 1990, p 96.
17 Speck B, Gluckman E, Haak HL, van Rood JJ: Treatment of aplastic anemia by antilymphocyte globulin with and without allogeneic bone marrow infusion. Lancet 1977;ii:1145.
18 Storb R, Erzioni R, Anasetti C, Appelbaum FR, Buckner CD, Besinger W, Bryant E, Clift R, Deeg HJ, Doney K, Flowers M, Hansen J, Martin P, Pepe M, Sale G, Sanders J, Singer J, Sullivan KM, Thomas ED, Witerspoon RP: Cyclophosphamide combined with antithymocyte globulin in preparation for allogeneic marrow transplants in patients with aplastic anemia. Blood 1994;84:941–949.
19 Socié G, Henry-Amar M, Cosset JM, Devergie A, Girinsky T, Gluckman E: Increased incidence of solid malignant tumors after bone marrow transplantation for severe aplastic anemia. Blood 1991;78:277–279.
20 Socié G, Amar MH, Bacigalupo A, Hows J, Tichelli A, Ljungman P, McCann S, Frickhofen N, van't Veer Korthof E, Gluckman E: Malignancies occurring after treatment of aplastic anemia: A survey conducted by the severe aplastic anaemia Working Party of the European Group for Bone Marrow Transplantation. N Engl J Med 1993;329:1152–1157.

Acta Haematologica

Acta Haematol 2000;103:26–32

# Results of Immunosuppression in Aplastic Anaemia

Judith C.W. Marsh

Department of Haematology, St. George Hospital Medical School, London, UK

**Key Words**
Antithymocyte globulin · Aplastic anaemia · Immunosuppression

**Abstract**
The availability of immunosuppressive agents, such as antilymphocyte globulin and cyclosporin, has had a major impact on the outcome of patients with aplastic anaemia. The majority of patients will show a response to immunosuppressive therapy. For those who fail to respond to an initial course, a second or further courses of immunosuppression can be given. Improvement in survival may also be due to the improved quality of supportive care available today for patients with aplastic anaemia. The additional use of haemopoietic growth factors such as granulocyte colony stimulating factor with immunosuppressive therapy requires further prospective randomised studies in order to evaluate whether they are of benefit for patients with aplastic anaemia. Because of the rarity of this condition, the use of multicentre prospective randomised studies is crucial for further evaluation of treatment modalities in aplastic anaemia.



## Introduction: Development of Antithymocyte Globulin for the Treatment of Aplastic Anaemia

Prior to the availability of antithymocyte globulin (ATG) and bone marrow transplantation (BMT) as therapeutic tools to treat patients with aplastic anaemia (AA), 50% of patients with AA died within 4–6 months [1]. Now for the majority, AA can be 'cured' or treated with allogeneic BMT or immunosuppressive therapy (IST), namely ATG and cyclosporin, respectively [2]. Most patients are not eligible for BMT and are treated with IST. Improvements in response rates and survival of patients treated with IST over the last three decades are probably multifactorial, including the additional use of cyclosporin with ATG, increasing use of multiple courses of ATG and improvements in supportive care.

In the late 1960s, Mathé et al. [3] used antilymphocyte globulin (ALG) as part of the conditioning regimen for BMT and noted a beneficial effect in some patients with AA [3]. Speck and Kissling [4, 5] in Basel used experimental rabbit models of benzene- and $^{32}$P-induced marrow aplasia in rabbits, and demonstrated that ALG and mismatched bone marrow could rescue them from aplasia. Subsequent clinical trials in humans showed that the marrow infusion was unnecessary for autologous haematological recovery after ATG therapy [6].

KARGER
Fax +41 61 306 12 34
E-Mail karger@karger.ch
www.karger.com


0001–5792/00/1031–0026$17.50/0

Accessible online at:
www.karger.com/journals/aha

Dr. J.C.W. Marsh
Department of Haematology
St. George's Hospital Medical School
Cranmer Terrace, London SW17 ORE (UK)
Tel. +44 181 725 3545, Fax +44 181 725 0245

## The Initial Clinical Studies of ATG in AA in Europe

The first clinical study of ATG as specific treatment for AA was in 29 patients treated with either ATG alone or ATG followed by infusion of haploidentical bone marrow, from centres in Basel, Paris and Leiden [6]. A response was seen in 12/29 and 50% of patients survived with a follow-up of up to 4.5 years. There was no significant difference in outcome between the two groups. The same group then initiated a larger prospective study comparing HLA-identical BMT with the use of ATG alone or in combination with HLA-haploidentical marrow [7]. Androgens were used routinely in patients in the two ATG arms. The survival of patients treated with ATG alone or with haploidentical bone marrow was 67 and 74%, respectively, and transfusion independence was achieved in 58 and 68%, respectively, by 8 months. The differences between the two ATG groups were not significant. This study highlighted (1) the delayed time to response after ATG, (2) the often incomplete recovery of blood counts after ATG compared with allogeneic BMT, (3) confirmed that infusion of haploidentical bone marrow was not necessary with ATG , and (4) demonstrated improvement in survival of AA patients, which was at least as good as for patients receiving an allogeneic BMT.

## Comparison of ATG with Supportive Care or with Androgens

The efficacy of ATG in the treatment of AA was confirmed by Champlin et al. [8], who performed the first prospective randomised trial comparing ATG with supportive care in 42 patients with severe and non-severe AA. In the ATG group, 11/21 (52%) patients responded by 3 months compared with none in the control arm. 12/21 control patients who survived for 3 months then went on to receive a course of ATG and 6 responded within 3 months. The overall actuarial survival of patients at 2 years was 41%, but 100% for responders compared with only 14% for non-responders.

A second prospective randomised study compared ATG with androgens in 44 patients with severe and non-severe AA. There were no responders among patients treated with androgens but 28% of ATG-treated patients became transfusion independent at 3 months [9].

## Use of ATG with Androgens

During the 1970s and early 1980s, the use of androgens with ATG had become routine in many centres, although their role was not clearly defined [10–13]. Several groups examined the impact of androgens on ATG treatment in studies comparing the combination of ATG and androgens with either androgens alone or ATG alone. A prospective randomised trial of ATG and androgens (with HLA-haploidentical bone marrow) compared with androgens alone was performed in 42 newly diagnosed patients with severe AA [14]. Significantly superior response and survival were observed in the ATG arm: 76% of patients survived at 2 years compared with 31% in the androgen arm. A small German study demonstrated improved response in patients with severe and non-severe AA among patients receiving the combination of ATG and androgens (11/15) compared with 4/15 receiving ATG alone [15]. A second prospective randomised study of 53 patients with severe or non-severe AA showed no difference whether treated with ATG and androgens (42% response) or with ATG and placebo (44% response) [16].

Larger but retrospective European Cooperative Group for BMT (EBMT) trials of patients treated during the late 1970s had suggested a trend towards improved survival when ATG was used with androgens but failed to reach statistical significance [10]. A more recent, large, prospective randomised study from the EBMT has helped clarify this issue. This study compared 69 patients treated with the combination of ATG and androgens with 65 patients receiving ATG without androgens [17]. A significantly better response rate was seen in patients receiving ATG and androgens (56% compared with 40% for ATG alone) and particularly in females with neutrophil count $<0.5 \times 10^9/l$: 60% response compared with 20% for ATG alone. There was no significant difference in survival between the two groups (71% for ATG and androgens and 65% for ATG alone), reflecting the ability to rescue non-responders with a second course of ATG or BMT.

## Cyclosporin in the Treatment of AA

*Cyclosporin Compared with ATG*

Small studies performed during the 1980s suggested that cyclosporin alone was effective in some patients with AA who were either untreated or who had failed ATG therapy [18–20]. A large French cooperative group performed a prospective randomised study comparing cyclosporin alone with ATG alone in 119 newly diagnosed patients with severe AA and showed a response rate at 3 months of 11.6% in the cyclosporin arm compared with 16% in the ATG arm. Survival of patients was similar in both groups (88% versus 75%). From this study, it appeared that cyclosporin was as effective as ATG, but the response rates seen in both groups at 3 months were much lower than previously reported and patient numbers small. Furthermore, response was impossible to assess after 3 months because non-responders crossed over to receive the other treatment arm. An observation of major concern from this study was the high number of early infective deaths (n = 20) occuring during ATG therapy [21].

*The Use of Cyclosporin in Combination with ATG*

A significant increase in response to IST among patients with severe and non-severe AA was observed in a prospective randomised multicentre German study comparing the combination of ATG and cyclosporin (43 patients) with ATG without cyclosporin (41 patients) [22]. At 3 months, the response was 65% for ATG and cyclosporin compared with 39% for ATG, and at 6 months 70% and 46%, respectively. Significantly better blood counts were achieved among responders in the ATG and cyclosporin arm compared with responders in the ATG arm, and fewer relapses were seen in the ATG and cyclosporin treatment group. The survival of all patients at 41 months was comparable (64% and 58%, respectively), although there was a trend for better survival of severe AA patients treated with ATG and cyclosporin (80%) compared with 44% receiving ATG ($p = 0.077$). Later follow-up of patients in this study demonstrated no significant difference in response at 12 months (74% for ATG and cyclosporin compared with 59% for ATG), but more patients in the ATG arm needed another course of IST. In addition, the actuarial risk of relapse became similar, but relapses occurred later in the ATG with cyclosporin arm [23]. There was no difference in survival between the two groups with an even longer follow-up of up to 11 years, again reflecting the ability to rescue non-responders with another course of ATG [N. Frickhofen, pers. commun.].

A later retrospective, single-centre evaluation of the combination of ATG and cyclosporin demonstrated an excellent response rate of 67% at 3 months and 75% at 12 months with an actuarial survival of 86% at 1 year and 72% at 2 years. There was a much lower number of early infective deaths compared with previous studies which was not associated with routine use of granulocyte-colony-stimulating factor (G-CSF) [24].

*Comparison of the Combination of ATG and Cyclosporin with Cyclosporin Alone for the Treatment of Patients with Non-Severe AA*

A recent prospective, randomised, multicentre European study compared the combination of ATG and cyclosporin with cyclosporin alone in 115 patients with non-severe AA, as defined by neutrophils $\geq 0.5 \times 10^9/l$ and transfusion dependence [25]. The aim was to determine whether cyclosporin alone was as effective as the current best regimen for severe AA. The combination of ATG and cyclosporin resulted in a significantly improved response rate (74%) at 6 months compared with 57% for cyclosporin alone, and significantly higher median haemoglobin levels and platelet counts. More patients in the cyclosporin arm (25%) required a course of ATG before 6 months because of disease progression compared with only 6% in the ATG and cyclosporin arm. The survival probabilities were identical (91% versus 93%), but the failure-free survival (excluding patients because of death, second treatment due to no response, disease progression or relapse) was 90% in the ATG and cyclosporin group compared with only 67% in the cyclosporin group. The study concluded that the combination of ATG and cyclosporin was superior to cyclosporin alone for patients with non-severe AA who are transfusion dependent in terms of response, quality of response, and requirement for a second course of IST.

## The Role of Corticosteroids in Immunosuppressive Regimens for AA

During the 1970s, the use of high-dose methylprednisolone (HDMP) was reported to be effective in some patients with AA [10, 26]. This led to the widespread practice of incorporating HDMP into ATG regimens, in the absence of controlled studies demonstrating a benefit in terms of response or survival. Furthermore, there were concerns about the short- and long-term toxicity of high doses of corticosteroids, particularly the risk of avascular necrosis as well as the increased risk of fungal and serious bacterial infections [27]. Doney et al. [28] reported no difference in response or survival for patients treated with ATG, androgens and low-dose prednisolone (0.5 mg/kg/day) compared with patients receiving ATG, androgens and HDMP (4.2 mg/kg/day), in a prospective randomised study of 68 patients with severe and non- severe AA [28]. The routine use of HDMP with ATG has now been abandoned, and there is no role for the use of corticosteroids alone as specific therapy for AA [2].

## The Use of G-CSF with Immunosuppressive Therapy

The rationale for designing protocols using G-CSF in combination with ATG and cyclosporin was as follows: (1) G-CSF might provide protection for neutropenic AA patients after administration of ATG during the 3 months before response was expected, and the French study had reported a high incidence of infective deaths during the first 3 months of ATG therapy [20]; (2) Bacigalupo et al. [29] had shown that large numbers of bone marrow progenitor cells could be mobilised following treatment with ATG, cyclosporin and daily G-CSF, and these progenitors might be important for re-seeding the bone marrow after IST and contribute to haematological recovery, and (3) studies had shown that G-CSF could correct the dysfunction of AA stem cells in vitro [30].

A pilot study of ATG, cyclosporin and 3 months of G-CSF in 40 patients with severe AA showed an apparent improvement in response of 82% at 3 months with an actuarial survival of 92%, with a maximum follow-up of almost 3 years [31]. This study was followed by a prospective, randomised, European multicentre trial of 102 patients comparing ATG, cyclosporin and G-CSF with ATG and cyclosporin alone. Although patients in the G-CSF arm had significantly fewer serious infections and more rapid neutrophil recovery, there was no significant difference in response rate (77.5% versus 81% at 6 months) or survival between the two groups [32].

There is concern that the chronic use of G-CSF in patients with AA may increase the risk of myelodysplastic syndrome and acute myelogenous leukaemia (MDS/AML). Between 5–15% of patients treated with IST are at risk of later MDS/AML [33–35]. It is not known whether this is a reflection of the natural history of AA and/or whether IST contributes to this risk. From the European study, to date, there appears to be no increased risk of MDS/AML but longer follow-up is required [31]. There was one case of MDS reported, however, a recent update of this study in 1998 revealed 4 cases of MDS/AML among 100 patients [A. Bacigalupo, pers. commun.]. Reports from Japan suggest an association between long duration or high doses of G-CSF therapy and risk of MDS/AML in children and adults treated with cyclosporin and G-CSF. One study in children [36] reported 11 cases of MDS/AML out of 167: no cases occurred among those treated with cyclosporin or G-CSF alone or with BMT, but the cases were observed exclusively in those treated with the combination of cyclosporin and G-CSF (11/50) giving a cumulative incidence of 47% at 6 years. In all cases, G-CSF was used at high dose (>10 μg/kg/day) and/or for more than 1 year. Monosomy 7 was detected in 10/11 cases. A second study from Japan in adult patients reported an incidence of MDS of 8.3% in the second year and 38.9% in the third year after treatment with G-CSF and cyclosporin with or without ATG [37].

At present, there is no indication for the routine chronic use of G-CSF after ATG, as a significant benefit in terms of response, and survival has not yet been demonstrated. Furthermore, the cost implications of using G-CSF for 3 months need to be carefully considered, and future controlled studies of haemopoietic growth factors used as part of the treatment of AA need to incorporate formal cost-benefit analyses.

## The Use of Repeated Courses of ATG

It is possible to administer two or more courses of ATG for either non-response to or relapse after an initial course of therapy. The risk of relapse after ATG is around 35% and appears to be higher for those who respond early compared with slow responders [38]. In some cases, it has been associated with cyclosporin withdrawal, and may sometimes respond to re-introduction of cyclosporin. If not, a second course of ATG would be appropriate. For the second course, it is possible to use either an alternative animal source of ATG (rabbit ATG, thymoglobulin) or to retreat with horse ATG [39]. Tichelli et al. [40] reported 43 severe AA patients who were retreated with horse ATG for failure to respond or relapse. 63% responded to the second horse ATG and this was well tolerated with no significant increase in side effects although serum sickness occurred earlier after repeated course compared with one course of ATG. The benefit of giving a second course of ATG was further emphasised by the survival of non-responders of a first course who went on to receive a second course (survival 55%) compared with 0% for non-responders who were not retreated with ATG. The use of multiple courses of IST was previously reported to be associated with an increased risk of clonal disorders such as MDS, AML and paroxysmal nocturnal haemoglobinuria (PNH), but the study by Tichelli failed to demonstrate a significant difference between patients receiving a single or multiple courses of ATG.

## Response to ATG in Patients with an Abnormal Clone

It is recognised that patients with AA may, not uncommonly, have a coexisting clone. This may be either a PNH clone occurring in the absence of haemolysis and demonstrated by flow-cytometric analysis of phospatidylinositol glycan (PIG)-anchored proteins, or an abnormal cytogenetic clone in the absence of haematological evidence of MDS or AML. A PNH clone may occur in 15–50% of AA patients [41, 42]. One study reported that response to IST was significantly lower compared with AA patients lacking a PNH clone [41]. In contrast, a second study of 11 AA patients showed no difference in response or survival among 17 patients with a PNH clone compared with AA patients with normal PIG-anchored protein expression [43].

In 4–11% of AA patients an abnormal cytogenetic clone can be demonstrated at diagnosis, most commonly trisomy 8 or 6 and anomalies of chromosomes 5 or 7 [44–46]. Often the abnormal clone is small in size, similar to the PNH clone when it coexists with normal cells. A small single-centre study of 13 AA patients with an abnormal cytogenetic clone demonstrated responses in all cases to one or more courses of IST, and no transformation to MDS/AML after a median follow-up of 4.1 years (range 1.2–11.2) [47]. In 4 patients, the cytogenetic clone disappeared after treatment, an observation previously reported by Mikhaelova et al. [46].

From these observations, the presence of a PNH clone or cytogenetic clone does not appear to affect the chance of response to IST. Further follow-up of these and more patients is needed to determine the long-term outcome of their disease, but so far, the use of IST does not appear to increase their risk of transformation or the size of the respective clone.

## ATG Therapy at the Extremes of Age

*Children*

Results of outcome of children with AA treated with IST have been variable [48–50]. Locascuilli et al. [50], on behalf of the EBMT in 1990, reported that the outcome depended primarily on disease severity with 37% survival for children with neutrophils $<0.2 \times 10^9/l$ compared with 56% for neutrophils $>0.2 \times 10^9/l$. ATG was used alone or in combination with androgens in this study. A more recent analysis by the same group, of 347 children, of whom 83% had severe AA (neutrophils $<0.5 \times 10^9/l$), showed that survival has improved significantly over time: 29% survival for children treated before 1980, 43% between 1980 and 1989, and 59% after 1990 [51]. Analysis of only those children with severe AA showed corresponding survival figures of 33, 60 and 70%, respectively. Thus, with time, the effect of age and the impact of disease severity have become less significant, as also seen in adults receiving IST [52].

*Elderly Patients*

Compared with allogeneic BMT for AA, it has been more difficult to set an upper age limit for ATG therapy. In elderly patients, there are natural concerns about the increased immediate risks of prolonged pancytopenia, particularly if there are coexisting serious medical problems, in addition to the concerns about an increased risk of clonal disorders. There has been only one study evaluating the effectiveness of IST in elderly patients [53]. This was a large retrospective multicentre EBMT analysis of 810 patients reported between 1974 and 1997. Most patients were treated with ATG alone or in combination with cyclosporin. Patients were evaluated according to age group: 127 of them were $\geq 60$ years of age (group 1) and 115 were 50–59 years (group 2). They were compared with 568 patients aged between 20 and 49 years (group 3). Response to IST, relapse rate and risk of clonal evolution were similar between all three age groups. Age was associated with an increased risk of death due to bleeding or infection and survival rates were 50%, 57% and 72% for patient groups 1, 2 and 3, respectively ($p < 0.001$). Thus, response was independent of age, but treatment was associated with increased mortality in elderly patients. The authors of this study concluded that treatment is feasible and there is no indication to withhold treatment solely because of age. Instead, the decision to use ATG should be determined by the general medical condition of the individual patient rather than her or his age alone.

## Improvement in Outcome with Time after Immunosuppressive Therapy

The results of IST in AA have improved greatly with time. A recent analysis by the EBMT of 1,182 patients treated with IST has shown a significant improvement in survival from 58% to 75% at 5 years over the last two decades, with an average reduction in mortality rate of 6% per year [52]. This may relate to the use of new immunosuppressive drugs such as cyclosporin with ATG compared with the use of ATG alone, improved supportive care and the use of repeated courses of ATG. The impact of G-CSF with ATG and cyclosporin, or used alone to treat serious infections, on improved outcome of patients needs further formal evaluation. Outcome is influenced by disease severity, particularly neutrophil count [11, 12, 52], although this may now be a less significant factor than previously reported [A. Bacigalupo, pers. commun.]. Because of factors such as continuing improvements in supportive care of AA patients with time, prospective randomised trials are vital for future studies of IST in AA. Follow-up of patients over many years and quality of life assessment are now even more relevant as more patients are surviving longer, and the risk and significance of later clonal disease, or small clonal populations in the absence of haematological evidence of pre-leukaemic or leukaemic transformation or haemolytic PNH, can be evaluated further.

## References


1 Lynch RE, Williams DM, Reading JC, Cartwright GE: The prognosis in aplastic anaemia. Blood 1975;45:517–528.

2 Young NS, Barrett AJ: The treatment of severe acquired aplastic anaemia. Blood 1995;85: 3367–3377.

3 Mathe G, Amiel JL, Schwarzenberg L, et al: Bone marrow grafts in man after conditioning by antilymphocyte serum. Br Med J 1970;i: 131–136.

4 Speck B, Kissling M: Successful bone marrow grafts in experimental aplastic anaemia using antilymphocyte serum for conditioning. Eur J Clin Biol Res 1971;10:1047–1051.

5 Speck B, Kissling M. Studies on bone marrow transplantation in experimental $^{32}$P-induced aplastic anaemia after conditioning with antilymphocyte serum. Acta Haematol 1973;50: 193–199.

6 Speck B, Gluckman E, Haak HL, et al: Treatment of aplastic anaemia by antilymphocyte globulin with and without allogeneic bone marrow infusions. Lancet 1977;ii:1145–1148.

7 Speck B, Gratwohl A, Nissen C, et al: Treatment of severe aplastic anaemia with antilymphocyte globulin or bone marrow transplantation. Br Med J 1981;282:860–863.

8 Champlin R, Ho W, Gale RP: Antilymphocyte globulin in patients with aplastic anaemia. N Engl J Med 1983;308:113–118.

9 Young N, Griffith P, Brittain E, et al: A multicentre trial of antithymocyte globulin in aplastic anaemia and related diseases. Blood 1988; 72:1861–1869.

10 Gluckman E, Devergie A, Poros A, et al: Results of immunosuppression in 170 cases of severe aplastic anaemia. Br J Haematol 1982; 51:541–550.

11 Speck B, Gratwohl A, Nissen C, et al: Treatment of severe aplastic anaemia. Exp Haematol 1986;14:126–132.

12 Marsh JCW, Hows JM, Bryett KA, et al: Survival after antilymphocyte globulin therapy for aplastic anaemia depends on disease severity. Blood 1987;70:1046–1052.

13 Bacigalupo A, Hows J, Gluckman E, et al: Bone marrow transplantation (BMT) versus immunosuppression for the treatment of severe aplastic anaemia (SAA): A report of the EBMT SAA Working Party. Br J Haematol 1988;70: 177–182.

14 Camitta B, O'Reilly R, Sensenbrenner L, et al: Antithoracic duct lymphocyte globulin therapy of severe aplastic anaemia. Blood 1983;62: 883–888.

15 Kaltwasser JP, Dix U, Schalk KP, et al: Effect of androgens on the response to antithymocyte globulin in patients with aplastic anaemia. Eur J Haematol 1988;40:111–118.

16 Champlin RE, Ho W, Feig SA, et al: Do androgens enhance the response to antithymocyte globulin in patients with aplastic anaemia? A prospective randomised trial. Blood 1985;66: 184–188.

17 Bacigalupo A, Chapple M, Hows J, et al: Treatment of aplastic anaemia (AA) with antilymphocyte globulin (ALG) and methylprednisolone (MPred) with or without androgens: A randomised trial from the EBMT SAA Working Party. Br J Haematol 1993;83:145–151.

18 Jacobs P, Wood L, Martell RW: Cyclosporin A in the treatment of severe acute aplastic anaemia. Br J Haematol 1985;61:267–272.

19 Leonard EM, Raefsky E, Griffith P, et al: Cyclosporine therapy of aplastic anaemia, congenital and acquired red cell aplasia. Br J Haematol 1989;72:278–284.

20 Hinterberger-Fischer M, Hocker P, Lechner K, et al: Oral cyclosporin-A is effective treatment for untreated and also for previously immunosuppressed patients with severe bone marrow failure. Eur J Haematol 1989;43:136–142.

21 Gluckman E, Esperou-Bourdeau H, Baruchel A, et al: Multicentre randomised study comparing cyclosporine-A alone and antithymocyte globulin with prednisolone for treatment of severe aplastic anaemia. Blood 1992;79: 2540–2546.

22 Frickhofen N, Kaltwasser JP, Schrezenmeier H, et al: Treatment of aplastic anaemia with antilymphocyte globulin and methylprednisolone with or without cyclosporine. N Engl J Med 1991;324:1297–1303.

23 Frickhofen N: Antilymphocyte globulin and methylprednisolone with or without cyclosporine A for treatment of aplastic anaemia (updated results of a German randomised trial); in Raghavachar A, Schrezenmeier H, Frickhofen N (eds): Aplastic Anaemia, Current Perspectives on the Pathogenesis and Treatment. New York, Blackwell-MZV, 1993, pp 118–125.

24 Rosenfeld SJ, Kimball J, Vining D, et al: Intensive immunosuppression with antithymocyte globulin and cyclosporine for severe acquired aplastic anaemia. Blood 1995;85:3058–3065.

25 Marsh J, Schrezenmeier H, Marin P, et al: Prospective randomised multicentre study comparing cyclosporin alone versus the combination of antithymocyte globulin and cyclosporin for treatment of patients with nonsevere aplastic anaemia: A report from the European Blood and Marrow Transplant (EBMT) Severe Aplastic Anaemia Working Party. Blood 1999;93: 2191–2195.

26 Bacigalupo A, Giordano D, Van Lint M, et al: Bolus methylprednisolone in severe aplastic anaemia. N Engl J Med 1979;300:501.

27 Marsh JCW, Zomas A, Hows JM, et al: Avascular necrosis after treatment of aplastic anaemia with antilymphocyte globulin and high dose methylprednisolone. Br J Haematol 1993;84:731–734.

28 Doney K, Pepe M, Storb R, et al: Immunosuppressive therapy of aplastic anaemia: Results of a prospective, randomised trial of antithymocyte globulin (ATG), methylprednisolone and oxymetholone to ATG, very high dose methylprednisolone and oxymetholone. Blood 1992; 79:2566–2571.

29 Bacigalupo A, Piaggio G, Podesta M, et al: Collection of peripheral blood hematopoietic progenitors (PBHP) from patients with severe aplastic anaemia (SAA) after prolonged administration of granulocyte colony stimulating factor. Blood 1993;82:1410–1414.

30 Scopes J, Daly S, Atkinson R, et al: Aplastic anaemia: Evidence of dysfunctional bone marrow progenitor cells and the corrective effect of granulocyte colony stimulating factor in vitro. Blood 1996;87:3179–3185.

31 Bacigalupo A, Broccia G, Corda W, et al: Antilymphocyte globulin, cyclosporin and granulocyte colony stimulating factor in patients with acquired severe aplastic anaemia (SAA): A pilot study of the EBMT SAA Working Party. Blood 1995;85:1348–1353.

32 Gluckman E, Rokicka-Milewska R, Gordon-Smith EC, et al: Results of a randomised study of glycosylated rHuGCSF Lenograstim in severe aplastic anaemia. Blood 1998; 92 (suppl 1):1551a.

33 Tichelli A, Gratwohl A, Wursch A, et al: Long term haematological complications in severe aplastic anaemia. Br J Haematol 1988;69:413–418.
34 De Planque M, Bacigalupo A, Wursch A, et al: Long term follow up of severe aplastic anaemia treated with antilymphocyte globulin. Severe Aplastic Anaemia Working Party of the European Cooperative Group for BMT (EBMT). Br J Haematol 1989; 73:121–126.
35 Socie G, Henry AM, Bacigalupo A, et al: Malignant tumours occurring after treatment of aplastic anaemia. EBMT SAAWP. N Engl J Med 1993;329:1152–1157.
36 Ohara A, Kojima S, Hamajima N, et al: Myelodysplastic syndrome and acute myelogenous leukaemia as a late clonal complication in children with acquired aplastic anaemia. Blood 1997;90:1009–1013.
37 Kaito K, Kobayashi M, Katayama T, et al: Long term administration of G-CSF for aplastic anaemia is closely related to the early evolution of monosomy 7 MDS in adults. Br J Haematol 1998;103:297–303.
38 Schrezenmeier H, Marin P, Raghavachar A, et al: Relapse of aplastic anaemia after immunosuppressive treatment: A report from the European Bone Marrow Transplantation Group SAA Working Party. Br J Haematol 1993;85: 371–377.
39 Marsh JCW, Gordon-Smith EC: Treatment options in severe aplastic anaemia. Lancet 1998; 351:1830–1831.
40 Tichelli A, Passweg J, Nissen C, et al: Repeated treatment with horse antilymphocyte globulin for severe aplastic anaemia. Br J Haematol 1998;100:393–400.
41 Schrezenmeier H, Hertenstein B, Wagner B, et al: A pathogenetic link between aplastic anaemia and paroxysmal nocturnal haemoglobinuria is suggested by a high frequency of aplastic anaemia patients with a deficiency of phosphatidylinositol glycan anchored proteins. Exp Haematol 1995;23:81–87.
42 Tooze JA, Saso R, Marsh JCW, et al: The novel monoclonal antibody By114 helps detect the early emergence of a paroxysmal nocturnal hemoglobinuria clone in aplastic anaemia. Exp Haematol 1995;23:1484–1491.
43 DeLord C, Tooze JA, Saso R, et al: Deficiency of glycosylphosphatidyl inositol-anchored proteins in patients with aplastic anaemia does not affect response to immunosuppressive therapy. Br J Haematol 1998;101:90–93.
44 Appelbaum F, Barrall J, Storb R, et al: Clonal cytogenetic abnormalities in patients with otherwise typical aplastic anaemia. Exp Haematol 1987;15:1134–1139.
45 Tichelli A, Socie G, Marsh J, et al: Cytogenetic abnormalities in aplastic anaemia. Bone Marrow Transplant 1996;7(suppl 1):268a.
46 Mikhailova N, Semareyo M, Fuhazza G, et al: Cytogenetic abnormalities in patients with severe aplastic anaemia. Haematologica 1996;81: 418–422.
47 Geary CG, Harrison CJ, Philpott NJ, et al: Abnormal cytogenetic clones in patients with aplastic anaemia: Response to immunosuppressive therapy. Br J Haematol 1999;104: 271–274.
48 Matloub YH, Bostrom B, Golembe B, et al: Antithymocyte globulin, cyclosporin and prednisolone for the treatment of severe aplastic anaemia in children. Am J Paediatr Haematol Oncol 1994;16:104–106.
49 Doney K, Leisenring W, Storb R, et al: Primary treatment of acquired aplastic anaemia: Outcomes with bone marrow transplantation and immunosuppressive therapy. Ann Intern Med 1997;126:107–115.
50 Locasciulli A, Vant Veer L, Bacigalupo A, et al: Treatment with marrow transplantation or immunosuppression of childhood acquired severe aplastic anaemia: A report from the EBMT SAA Working Party. Bone Marrow Transplant 1990;6:211–217.
51 Locasciulli A: Treatment of children with acquired aplastic anaemia; in Schrezenmeier H, Bacigalupo A (eds): Aplastic Anaemia. Cambridge, Cambridge University Press, in press.
52 Bacigalupo A, Brand R, Socie G, et al: Bone marrow transplantation (BMT) or immunosuppressive therapy (IS) for patients with severe aplastic anaemia (SAA): A report of the European Group for Blood and Marrow Transplantation (EBMT). Blood 1998;92 (suppl 1): 637a.
53 Tichelli A, Socie G, Henry-Amar M, et al: Effectiveness of immunosuppressive therapy in older patients with aplastic anaemia. Ann Intern Med 1999;130:193–201.

Acta Hæmatologica

Acta Haematol 2000;103:33–40

# Cell Cycling Stress in the Monocyte Line as a Risk Factor for Progression of the Aplastic Anaemia/Paroxysmal Nocturnal Haemoglobinuria Syndrome to Myelodysplastic Syndrome

Catherine Nissen Alexander Genitsch Silvia Sendelov
Verena Dalle Carbonare Aleksandra Wodnar-Filipowicz

Department of Research and Department of Internal Medicine, Division of Haematology, University Hospital, Basel, Switzerland

**Key Words**
Antilymphocyte globulin treatment · Aplastic anaemia · Myelodysplastic syndrome · Paroxysmal nocturnal haemoglobinuria

**Abstract**
Severe aplastic anaemia (SAA) causes permanent stem cell damage from which patients do not recover after treatment with antilymphocyte globulin (ALG). To produce peripheral blood values compatible with life, the few remaining stem and precursor cells are put under stress. We defined a 'stress factor' (SF) for various haematopoietic lines as the ratio of the corresponding peripheral blood (PB) value to the total colony number in short-term bone marrow cultures from 86 patients with different outcomes. Both values are expressed as percentage of normal, hence SF averages 1 in normal steady-state haematopoiesis. SF was elevated in all patients, from 2-to 40-fold, with wide variations in different patient groups and striking differences between haematopoietic lineages. In long-term disease-free survivors after ALG (group 1) the mean total colony count was 19% of normal, with a significantly higher proportion of erythroid burst-forming units compared to normal. They had ineffective erythropoiesis with haemoglobin (Hb) values below, and reticulocyte counts above normal; platelet counts were 67% of normal. In contrast, monocyte counts were in the high normal range, resulting in a high SF (18.7 ± 1.9) for monocytes. In patients who developed paroxysmal nocturnal haemoglobinuria (PNH) after ALG (group 2), ineffective erythropoiesis, reflecting haemolysis, was more pronounced and they had striking relative monocytosis, resulting in a significantly higher SF for monocytes (33.7 ± 5.7) compared with group 1 ($p < 0.0001$). High monocyte counts most likely reflect the relative resistance of nucleated cells to complement, compared with red cells and platelets. Patients who developed myelodysplastic syndrome (MDS) or acute myeloid leukaemia (AML) after ALG, with or without PNH (group 3), had the highest SF for monocytes (39 ± 10). They also had neutrophil counts in the upper range, or above normal, resulting in a high SF for neutrophils: 32 ± 19. In patients with persisting or relapsing-remitting pancytopenia without a clinically detectable clonal disorder (group 4), all values were strikingly similar to those of the PNH group. In patients who achieved normal PB values after uncomplicated bone marrow transplantation (group 5), the SF averaged 3, but they also had ineffective erythropoiesis and mild relative monocytosis, a possible sign of occult PNH. We conclude that all patients after treatment of SAA have ineffective

KARGER
Fax + 41 61 306 12 34
E-Mail karger@karger.ch
www.karger.com


0001–5792/00/1031–0033$17.50/0

Accessible online at:
www.karger.com/journals/aha

Catherine Nissen, MD
Department of Research, University Hospital
CH–4031 Basel (Switzerland)
Tel. +41 61 265 23 33, Fax +41 61 265 23 50
E-Mail nissen@magnet.ch

erythropoiesis and relative monocytosis, and that these abnormalities probably reflect PNH. We suggest that the resulting high SF for the leukocyte – particularly the monocyte line – predisposes to the development of MDS/AML. We discuss how these results may provide some of the missing pieces in the puzzle of SAA/PNH.



## Introduction

After apparently successful immunosuppressive treatment of severe aplastic anaemia (SAA) with antilymphocyte globulin (ALG), improvement of peripheral blood (PB) values is not matched by a corresponding increase of precursor cells. Patients have a permanent loss of stem and precursor cells [1–8]. Line-specific haematopoietic cytokines, such as erythropoietin and G-CSF as well as the multilineage growth factor flt3 ligand, remain chronically elevated [9], indicating persistent endogenous stimulation at all maturation stages of haematopoiesis. Chronic overstimulation causes an increase in cycling rate leading to premature ageing, as documented by accelerated telomere shortening in these patients [10]. This probably explains why they are prone to developing myelodysplastic syndrome (MDS) and acute myelogenous leukaemia (AML) [11–13]. The intricate relationship between SAA and paroxysmal nocturnal haemoglobinuria (PNH) [14, 15], the high prevalence of clinically unrecognized PNH in SAA before and after treatment [14, 16–18], and the presence of the PNH clone even in normals [19] remain a puzzle. It is not known why PNH patients are at particularly high risk of developing MDS/AML [20].

During the early recovery phase after ALG, improvement of the platelet count and the haemoglobin (Hb) value lag behind the increase in leucocytes in the majority of patients. This difference is intriguing, and not compatible with the concept that SAA is a disease of primitive precursor cells only. In addition to the stem cell defect, there must be conditions in vivo which preferentially affect RBC and platelets. Macrocytosis and ineffective erythropoiesis during early recovery [21] and persistent thrombocytopenia associated with a 'shift to the left' of bone marrow (BM)-megakaryocytes [22] argues in favour of a pathology in the thrombo-erythroid line from which the myeloid line is apparently spared. Since the same lineage discrepancy is also observed in non-severe untreated AA, these abnormalities probably reflect AA-specific disease activity persisting after IST.

We compared BM colony-forming capacity with corresponding PB values in a large group of patients recovering from SAA after ALG and found that colony counts were low, as expected. We found that mild ineffective erythropoiesis persisted in all patients, including disease-free long-term survivors with PB values in the normal range, and that these abnormalities were paralleled by relative monocytosis. In PNH patients, ineffective erythropoiesis and relative monocytosis were more pronounced. We propose that this subtle lineage disbalance (1) is a sensitive indicator of subclinical PNH, and (2) shows that particular 'cycling stress' is imposed on the monocyte lineage, which may explain the high incidence of leukaemia in SAA/PNH.

## Patients and Methods

*Patients*

Included in the analysis were patients treated for SAA in a long-term single-centre cohort study at our hospital, in whom complete PB values and results of short-term BM cultures performed on the same day were available. A total of 499 examinations in 86 patients after treatment are the basis of the analysis. Five groups of patients were identified according to treatment (82 received ALG and 4, an allogenic BM graft from a matched sibling donor) and to treatment outcome as follows.

*Group 1.* 37 patients treated with ALG who achieved complete haematological remission (CR), defined as neutrophils $\geq 1.5 \times 10^9$/l, monocytes $\geq 0.12 \times 10^9$/l, reticulocytes $\geq 40 \times 10^9$/l, platelets $\geq 150 \times 10^9$/l and a Hb $\geq$ 12 g% for female and $\geq$13 g% for male patients, after a single course of ALG, and who neither developed PNH nor MDS/AML within 5 years after treatment.

*Group 2.* 12 ALG-treated patients who developed PNH after treatment, documented by clinical symptoms or subclinical signs of PNH, as described by Schrezenmeier et al. [23] and Socié and Gluckman [24] in this issue.

*Group 3.* 6 ALG patients who developed MDS/AML, according to the criteria of Socié and Gluckman [24] in this issue.

*Group 4.* 27 ALG patients who did not achieve CR or had relapsing/remitting AA but no evidence of either PNH or MDS/AML.

*Group 5.* 4 patients treated with bone marrow transplantation (BMT) from an HLA-matched sibling donor with a stable graft, normal PB values and no graft-versus-host disease.

*Methods*

*PB Analysis.* Standard haematological laboratory tests for neutrophil, monocyte, platelet, reticulocyte counts and Hb values were performed. Lymphocyte values were not included in the analysis.

*BM Cultures.* Short-term BM cultures in methylcellulose were performed as described [25]. A human leucocyte-conditioned medium with standard activity was used for stimulation. The colony read-out at 2 weeks was done by one person.

*Calculation of 'Haematopoietic Stress Factor'.* We defined a 'stress factor' (SF) for various haematopoietic lines as the ratio of the corresponding PB value to the total colony number in short-term BM

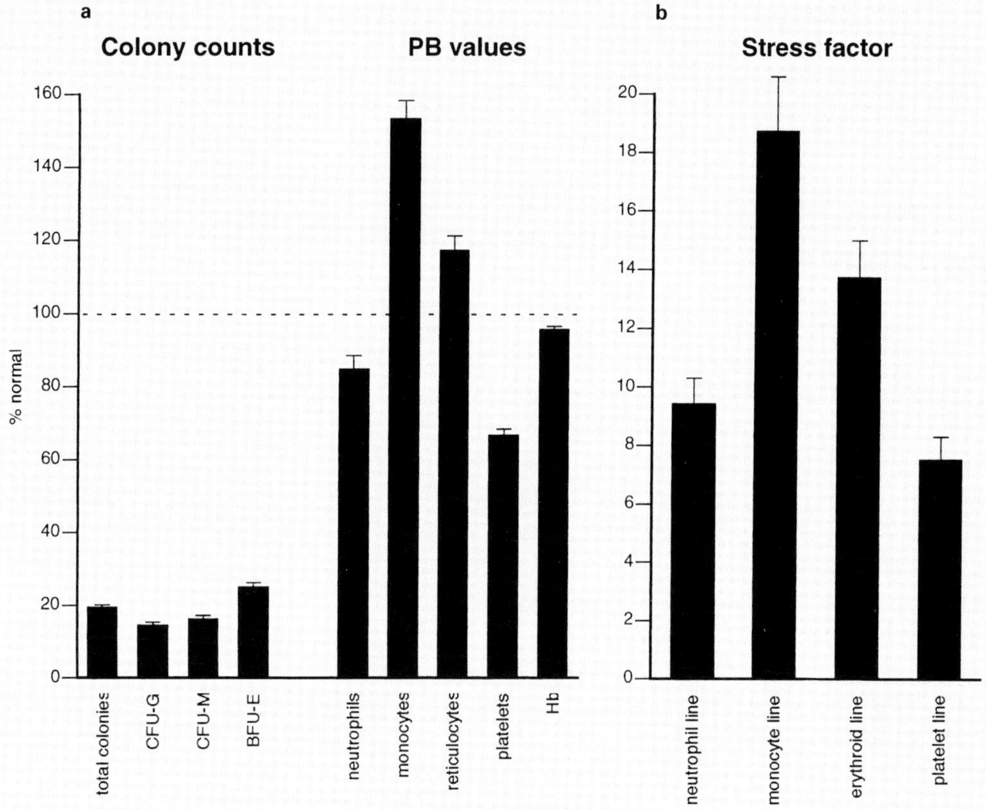


**Fig. 1.** Colony counts, PB values and SF in group 1 ('good risk'). Colony counts and PB values are given in percent of normal and SF was calculated as described in 'Methods'.

cultures. Both values are expressed as percentages of normal. Normal PB values were obtained from 30 male and 30 female blood donors (mean ± SEM): neutrophils 3.59 ± 0.15 × $10^9$/l, monocytes 0.34 ± 0.01 × $10^9$/l, reticulocytes 50.4 ± 2.1 × $10^9$/l, platelets 257 ± 7.9 × $10^9$/l, Hb in males 14.7 ± 0.2 g%, in females 13.0 ± 0.1 g%. Normality for colony numbers was established in 45 normal donors for BMT. Mean total colonies per 2 × $10^5$ nucleated cells were 150 ± 8 (CFU-G 36 ± 3, CFU-M 53 ± 3 and BFU-E 61 ± 6). Under physiological conditions, SF equals 1 on average, while any value over 1 reflects a relative deficit in precursor cells compared with their progeny circulating in PB.

## Results and Discussion

The haematological 'stress' resulting from few stem cells providing progeny compatible with life was calculated for SAA patients after treatment. Results were grouped according to clinical criteria.

### *'Good Risk' Patients (Group 1)*

In figure 1 we show results of patients who are in CR after a single course of ALG and who did not develop a clonal haematological disorder within at least 5 years after treatment. The sucrose test on RBC for detection of PNH, the Coombs' test for detection of anti-RBC autoantibodies, iron excretion in the urine as a sign of intravascular haemolysis and FACS analysis for the detection of PB cells lacking GPI-linked proteins were performed yearly; the results were always negative.

In this 'good risk' group, the mean total colony count was 19% of normal with little variation, confirming persisting stem cell damage common to all patients achieving apparent remission after ALG. Compared to normal, the proportion of BFU-E was significantly higher than that of CFU-GM, and CFU-M were particularly scarce. This inverted BFU-E to CFU-GM ratio suggests preferential

**Table 1.** Colony counts in BM cultures and PB values after treatment of SAA in different patient groups in percent of normal (mean ± SEM)

| Patient group | Patients/ examinations | BM colonies | | | | PB values | | | | |
|---|---|---|---|---|---|---|---|---|---|---|
| | | total | CFU-G | CFU-M | BFU-E | neutrophils | monocytes | reticulocytes | platelets | Hb |
| Group 1 | 37/226 | 19.3±0.9 | 14.5±0.9 | 16.2±1.2 | 25.0±1.3 | 84.7±3.9 | 153.3±5.2 | 117.2±4.1 | 66.6±1.9 | 95.7±1.0 |
| Group 2 | 12/92 | 11.0±1.2 | 11.1±1.6 | 7.5±1.3 | 14.3±1.5 | 49.9±4.1 | 111.2±9.3 | 157.3±11.2 | 46.4±3.9 | 81.6±2.2 |
| Group 3 | 6/32 | 10.3±2.2 | 9.1±2.2 | 10.8±3.7 | 11.1±2.0 | 63.2±12.8 | 110.9±12.4 | 140.2±16.2 | 54.4±7.2 | 82.0±2.8 |
| Group 4 | 27/142 | 14.0±1.7 | 13.7±1.9 | 13.2±2.5 | 15.2±1.8 | 66.9±5.6 | 118.7±7.2 | 111.8±4.7 | 46.6±3.3 | 81.1±1.6 |
| Group 5 | 4/7 | 48.0±1.8 | 53.9±15.7 | 35.7±8.2 | 55.0±15.7 | 114.9±32.6 | 151.9±20.0 | 125.1±22.8 | 86.4±7.6 | 100.9±2.5 |

differentiation from uncommitted precursor cells towards the erythroid line, reflecting peripheral requirements, e.g. following loss of mature RBC. This is supported by a significant difference between reticulocyte counts and Hb values ($p < 0.0001$). Although BFU-E were relatively high, Hb values were below normal (96%). In contrast, monocyte counts were above normal (153%), although CFU-M numbers were particularly low. Neutrophils were 85% and platelet counts were 67% of normal. The resulting SF (fig. 1b) was higher for the monocyte line than for all the other lineages ($p < 0.0001$).

How can ineffective erythropoiesis, mild thrombocytopenia and relative monocytosis – the combination of abnormalities found in these patients – be linked together? In the absence of anti-erythrocyte autoantibodies, ineffective erythropoiesis reflects otherwise unexplained haemolysis and thus – in the context of SAA – probably PNH. The relatively high monocyte counts – which could not be explained by increased peripheral requirements, since the patients were in good clinical condition without signs of infection and were not treated with G-CSF or GM-CSF – could be explained by their in vivo resistance to complement. Assuming that these patients had a small population of PNH erythrocytes, as evidenced by ineffective erythrocytosis, it is likely that part of their monocytes also had the PNH defect. Monocytes missing GPI-linked proteins are known to be more resistant to complement lysis than red cells and platelets: as nucleated cells with a functional DNA-RNA machinery, they can react to complement attack with de novo synthesis of regulatory proteins and are thus better protected than non-nucleated cells [26]. (Lymphocyte counts which we do not show here were also relatively high, probably for the same reason.) To sum up: the combination of mild thrombocytopenia/anaemia with relative monocytosis is best explained by the presence of a population of multipotential haematopoietic cells giving rise to complement-sensitive progeny.

*Patients with Clinical Problems after ALG and Post-BMT Patients (Groups 2–5)*

In table 1 we show colony counts and PB values in patients with a less favourable outcome after ALG and in patients treated with BMT (groups 2–5), in comparison with group 1. The resulting SF values are shown in figure 2.

In patients who developed PNH after ALG, the mean total colony count was 11% of normal, with a more pronounced shift towards BFU-E than in patients of group 1. The corresponding PB values showed the classical PNH characteristics, i.e. anaemia with reticulocytosis. As in group 1, monocyte counts were comparatively high (111% of normal), probably reflecting the relative complement resistance of nucleated cells mentioned above. Platelet counts were 46% of normal, most likely due to their high sensitivity to complement as non-nucleated cells. Neutrophil counts were 50% of normal. The relatively high monocyte counts produced by the very low number of CFU-GM (7% of normal) resulted in a high stress factor for the monocyte line. It was 34 ± 6 compared to 19 ± 2 ($p < 0.0001$) in patients of group 1. Excessive stress of cycling in the leukocyte line – which has the highest cell turnover – is likely to contribute to leukaemogenesis in these patients.

From the comparison of results in group 1 and 2, it appears that ineffective erythropoiesis and relative monocytosis is common to all patients, whether they have clinical PNH or not. For the ultimate proof that this indicates the presence of the PNH clone, PCR analysis for mutations in the PIG-A gene would be required. However, relative monocytosis could be a very sensitive indicator of PNH. Since it is a measure of monocyte survival in vivo, it may be more sensitive than tests analysing cells ex vivo under non-physiological conditions. For the daily routine, we suggest that relative monocytosis in AA should draw attention to the possible presence of PNH cells.

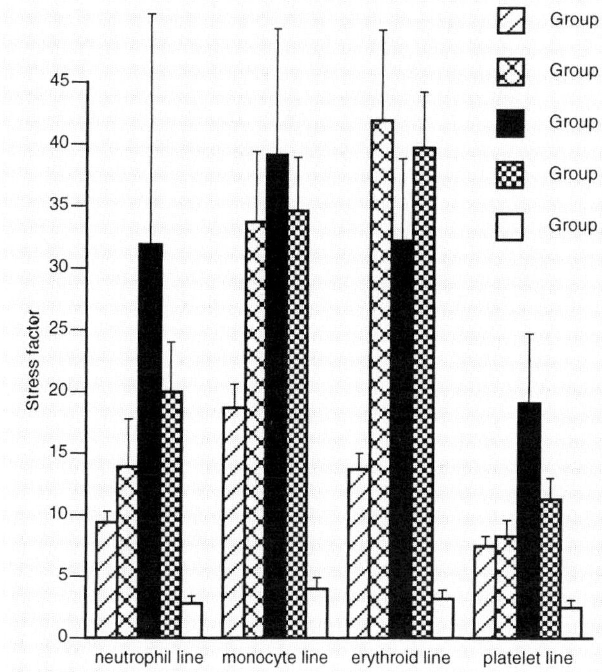


**Fig. 2.** SF for different haematopoietic lineages in patients with different clinical outcomes. Group 1: 'good risk'; group 2: developed laboratory or clinical PNH; group 3: developed MDS/AML with or without PNH; group 4: did not achieve CR or had relapsing/remitting aplasia without MDS/AML/PNH; group 5: achieved a stable haematopoietic graft with normal PB values.

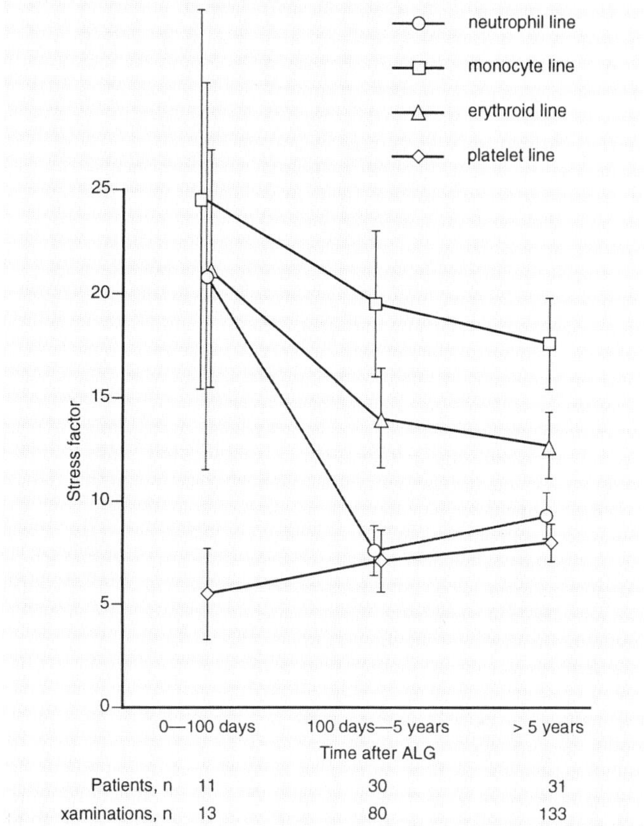


**Fig. 3.** Development over time of SF in group 1 ('good risk').

In patients who developed MDS/AML with or without PNH (group 3), the SF for the monocyte line was 39 ± 10, which was higher than in all other groups. In addition, the SF for the neutrophil line was higher than in all other patient groups (32 ± 19 versus 9 ± 1 in group 1). Thus, leukaemogenesis in these patients was indeed associated with a high SF for both the monocyte and the neutrophil line. Additionally forcing cell division in the neutrophil line with G-CSF can be potentially harmful and may be responsible for the increased incidence of AML in AA patients [27] and in patients with chronic severe neutropenia [28] undergoing long-term treatment with G-CSF.

In patients with an incomplete or transient response to ALG who did not develop a clonal disorder (group 4), colony counts were lower than in patients of group 1, as expected. Unexpectedly, however, a higher degree of ineffective erythopoiesis and relative monocytosis, i.e., the typical signs of PNH, were observed. Accordingly, 'cycling stress' values were very similar to those observed in PNH patients. This suggests that there is more clinically unrecognised PNH in patients with prolonged pancytopenia, in other words, that pancytopenia helps to 'hide' the PNH clone, i.e. that pancytopenia may be a reaction to PNH.

After BMT (group 5) colony counts did not reach normality (48% of normal) as described previously by us [29] and others [8], and the stress factor was increased accordingly. They also had mild ineffective erythropoiesis and relative monocytosis, which may reflect partial chimerism with some residual cells carrying PNH traits. The appropriate controls would be patients transplanted for diseases other than SAA, which were not done in this context.

*Long-Term Evolution of the Haematopoietic SF*

Because the stem cell defect after ALG is irreversible, cycling stress is bound to be permanent. The long-term follow-up of patients in group 1 is shown in figure 3. The

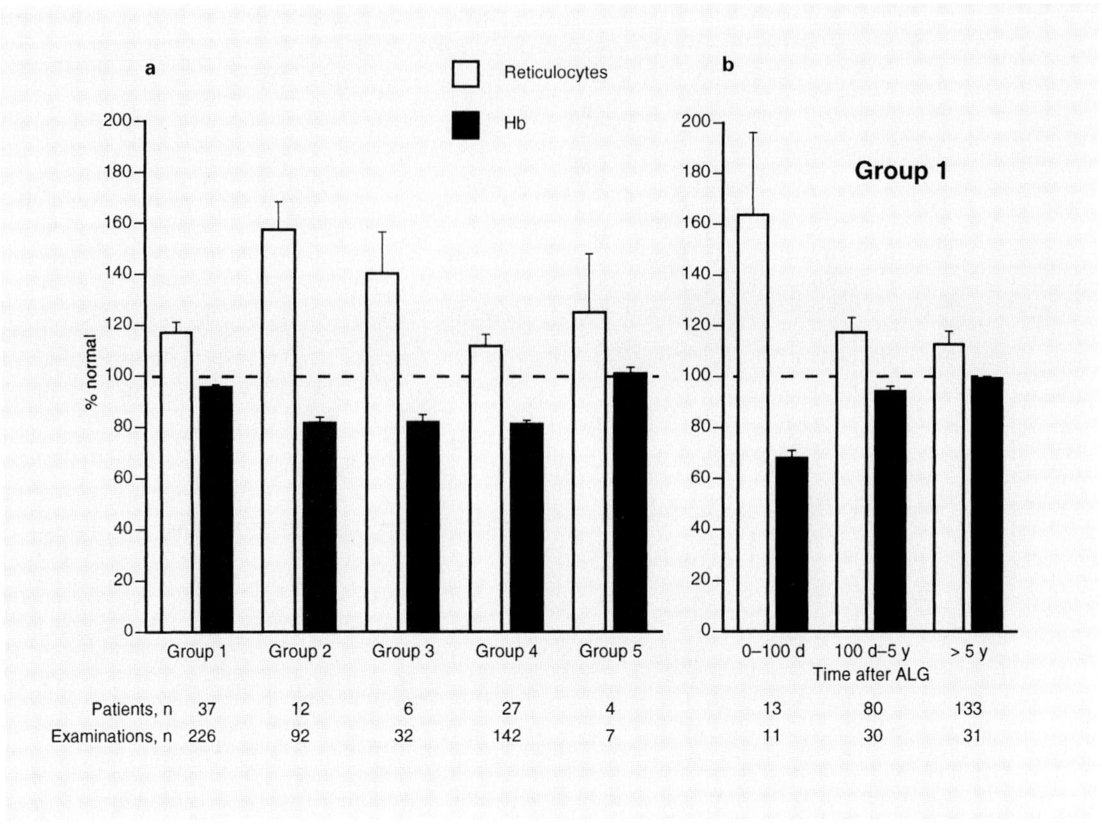


**Fig. 4.** **a** Ineffective erythropoiesis (reticulocytes versus Hb in % of normal) after treatment for SAA in different patient groups. Group 1: $p < 0.008$, group 2: $p < 0.0001$, group 3: $p < 0.0001$; group 4: $p < 0.0001$, group 5: n.s. **b** Values for group 1 at different time points.

discrepancy between colony counts and PB values, and thus the stress imposed on precursor cells was nearly 3 times as high for the neutrophil line during the first 3 months than thereafter, suggesting that there is particular vulnerability for the development of leukaemic clones during the early recovery phase. Therefore, adding G-CSF routinely to standard immunosuppressive treatment (IST) of SAA in patients who do not suffer from neutropenic bacterial infection may unnecessarily recruit large numbers of granulocytes, and thereby further increase the high cycling stress typical of the early post-ALG period.

*Ineffective Erythropoiesis as Sign of PNH*

Hb values were below, and reticulocyte counts were higher than normal in all patient groups, even after BMT, indicating haemolysis, as shown separately in figure 4. The difference was significant in all patients after ALG, showing that they have haemolysis, and thus probably PNH, whether clinically recognized or not.

This apparent omnipresence of PNH traits in patients after ALG raises speculations about the pathophysiological significance of PNH in normal and abnormal haematopoiesis. The PNH clone could be a substitute tissue within the aplastic marrow [15]. As an alternative explanation, we suggest that the primary expansion of the PNH clone is due to its relative resistance to apoptotic damage, and that AA is the result of the patient's immunological fight against the expanding abnormal clone. This hypothesis is largely based on existing knowledge. It is known that PNH precursor cells do not have a growth advantage over normal precursors [30]; they are, however, more resistant to Fas-induced apoptosis [31]. The following 'scenario' might unite these findings. Drugs, chemicals and viruses associated with AA cause mild transient pancytopenia in all patients. Apoptosis is known to be involved in the resulting cell damage. The normally present PNH clone, though having no growth advantage in vitro, may be more resistant to these toxic agents in vivo by virtue of its relative resistance to apoptosis-inducing agents, and therefore expand. The immune system recognising the abnormal clone will attempt to eradicate it. If PNH precursors share antigenic properties with their normal counterparts – which may be a rare incidence, but worth future research – the immune system would also recognize normal cells and destroy them as 'innocent bystanders'. The result would be successful eradication of PNH at the cost of the normal haematopoietic system, manifested clinically as very severe AA with high levels of cytokines, like IL-2 and IFNγ, reflecting an ongoing immune reaction, with no detectable PNH. In patients with a compromised immune system, on the other hand, the PNH clone will expand and produce near-normal PB values except for signs of haemolysis. In 'good risk' patients (group 1), ineffective erythropoiesis was most pronounced during the first 3 months after ALG, i.e., when patients were still immunosuppressed, suggesting that the compromised immune system allowed a complement-sensitive population of RBC to transiently expand.

Our previous finding that IL-2 release is low in PNH patients compared to AA patients not developing PNH [25] is in keeping with the role of the immune system in suppressing the PNH clone. The observation that the presence of a GPI-lacking clone before IST does not preclude a response, but that these patients have a high risk of later developing PNH [32] is compatible with our hypothesis: PNH cells present at the time of diagnosis of SAA indicate that the immune system failed to eradicate the abnormal clone, and also allowed its expansion after IST. The fact that PNH cells have a survival advantage in the SCID mouse [33] also argues in favour of this hypothesis. Should the hypothesis that an immunosuppressed environment favours the outgrowth of PNH be correct, the consequence for the clinic would be that immunosuppression in SAA should be limited to the minimum required to control the autoimmune reaction causing pancytopenia. To create a therapeutic cocktail tailored to knock out the cells that cause pancytopenia and to preserve immunocompetent cells fighting the PNH clone may be a goal of future research.

We conclude that the few residual precursor cells after ALG produce progeny characterised by ineffective erythropoiesis compatible with chronic haemolysis, and thus probably the permanent presence of PNH cells. The relative overproduction of leucocytes resulting from chronic haematopoietic stimulation, aiming primarily at normalisation of the Hb value, causes strong 'cycling stress' in the myeloid series and thereby probably contributes to leukaemogenesis.

## References


1 Juneja HS, Lee S, Gardner FH: Human long-term bone marrow cultures in aplastic anemia. Int J Cell Cloning 1989;7:129–135.
2 Fujiwara M: Long-term cultures of marrow cells from the patients with aplastic anemia. Nippon Ketsueki Gakkai Zasshi 1990;53:533–540.
3 Gibson FM, Gordon-Smith EC: Long-term culture of aplastic anaemia bone marrow. Br J Haematol 1990;75:421–427.
4 Bacigalupo A, Figari O, Tong J, Piaggio G, Miceli S, Frassoni F, Caciagli P, Badolati G, Marmont AM: Long-term marrow culture in patients with aplastic anemia compared with marrow transplant recipients and normal controls. Exp Hematol 1992; 20:425–430.
5 Nissen C, Wodnar-Filipowicz A, Slanicka-Krieger M, Gratwohl A, Tichelli A, Speck B: Persistent growth impairment of bone marrow stroma after antilymphocyte globulin treatment for severe aplastic anaemia and its association with relapse. Eur J Haematol 1995;55: 255–261.
6 Maciejewski JP, Selleri C, Sato T, Anderson S, Young NS: A severe and consistent deficit in marrow and circulating primitive hematopoietic cells (long-term culture-initiating cells) in acquired aplastic anemia. Blood 1996;88: 1983–1991.
7 Manz CY, Nissen C, Wodnar-Filipowicz A: Deficiency of CD34+ c-*kit*+ and CD34+38– hematopoietic precursors in aplastic anemia after immunosuppressive treatment. Am J Hematol 1996;52:264–274.
8 Podestà M, Piaggio G, Frassoni F, Pitto A, Zikos P, Sessarego M, Abate M, Teresa Van Lint M, Berisso G, Bacigalupo A: The assessment of the hematopoietic reservoir after immunosuppressive therapy or bone marrow transplantation in severe aplastic anemia. Blood 1998;91:1959–1965.
9 Wodnar-Filipowicz A, Lyman SD, Gratwohl A, Tichelli A, Speck B, Nissen C: Flt3 ligand level reflects hematopoietic progenitor cell function in aplastic anemia and chemotherapy-induced bone marrow aplasia. Blood 1996;88: 4493–4499.
10 Ball SE, Gibson FM, Rizzo S, Tooze JA, Marsh JC, Gordon-Smith EC: Progressive telomere shortening in aplastic anemia. Blood 1998;91: 3582–3592.
11 Tichelli A, Gratwohl A, Wursch A, Nissen C, Speck B: Late haematological complications in severe aplastic anaemia. Br J Haematol 1988; 69:413–418.
12 de Planque MM, Bacigalupo A, Wursch A, Hows JM, Devergie A, Frickhofen N, Brand A, Nissen C: Long-term follow-up of severe aplastic anaemia patients treated with antithymocyte globulin. Severe Aplastic Anaemia Working Party of the European Cooperative Group for Bone Marrow Transplantation (EBMT). Br J Haematol 1989;73:121–126.
13 Socié G, Henry-Amar M, Bacigalupo A, Hows J, Tichelli A, Ljungman P, McCann SR, Frickhofen N, Van't Veer-Korthof E, Gluckman E: Malignant tumors occurring after treatment of aplastic anemia. European Bone Marrow Transplantation-Severe Aplastic Anaemia Working Party. N Engl J Med 1993;329: 1152–1157.
14 Griscelli-Bennaceur A, Gluckman E, Scrobohaci ML, Jonveaux P, Vu T, Bazarbachi A, Carosella ED, Sigaux F, Socie G: Aplastic anemia and paroxysmal nocturnal hemoglobinuria: Search for a pathogenetic link. Blood 1995; 85:1354–1363.

15 Schrezenmeier H, Hertenstein B, Wagner B, Raghavachar A, Heimpel H: A pathogenetic link between aplastic anemia and paroxysmal nocturnal hemoglobinuria is suggested by a high frequency of aplastic anemia patients with a deficiency of phosphatidylinositol glycan anchored proteins [published erratum appears in Exp Hematol 1995 Feb;23(2):181]. Exp Hematol 1995;23:81–87.
16 Nissen C, Gratwohl A, Speck B, Würsch A, Moser Y, Weis J: Acquired aplastic anaemia: A PNH-like disease? Br J Haematol 1986;64: 355–362.
17 Nakakuma H, Nagakura S, Iwamoto N, Kawaguchi T, Hidaka M, Horikawa K, Kagimoto T, Shido T, Takatsuki K: Paroxysmal nocturnal hemoglobinuria clone in bone marrow of patients with pancytopenia. Blood 1995;85: 1371–1376.
18 Azenishi Y, Ueda E, Machii T, Nishimura J, Hirota T, Shibano M, Nakao S, Kinoshita T, Mizoguchi H, Kitani T: CD59-deficient blood cells and PIG-A gene abnormalities in Japanese patients with aplastic anaemia. Br J Haematol 1999;104:523–529.
19 Araten DJ, Nafa K, Pakdeesuwan K, Luzzatto L: Clonal populations of hematopoietic cells with paroxysmal nocturnal hemoglobinuria genotype and phenotype are present in normal individuals. Proc Natl Acad Sci USA 1999;96: 5209–5214.
20 Harris JW, Koscick R, Lazarus HM, Eshleman JR, Medof ME: Leukemia arising out of paroxysmal nocturnal hemoglobinuria. Leuk Lymphoma 1999;32:401–426.
21 Marsh JC, Hows JM, Bryett KA, Al-Hashimi S, Fairhead SM, Gordon-Smith EC: Survival after antilymphocyte globulin therapy for aplastic anemia depends on disease severity. Blood 1987;70:1046–1052.
22 Tichelli A, Gratwohl A, Nissen C, Signer E, Stebler Gysi C, Speck B: Morphology in patients with severe aplastic anemia treated with antilymphocyte globulin. Blood 1992;80:337–345.
23 Schrezenmeier H, Hildebrand A, Rojewski M, Häcker H, Heimpel H, Raghavachar A: Paroxysmal nocturnal haemoglobinuria: A replacement of haematopoietic tissue? Acta Haematol 2000;103:41–48.
24 Socié G, Gluckman E: Cure from severe aplastic anemia in vivo and late effects. Acta Haematol 2000;103:49–54.
25 Nissen C, Tichelli A, Gratwohl A, Warthmann C, Moser Y, dalle Carbonare V, Sendelov S, Chklovskaia E, Jansen W, Wodnar-Filipowicz A, Sadallah S, Speck B: High incidence of transiently appearing complement-sensitive bone marrow precursor cells in patients with severe aplastic anemia – A possible role of high endogenous IL-2 in their suppression. Acta Haematol 1999;101:165–172.
26 Morgan BP: Complement membrane attack on nucleated cells: Resistance, recovery and nonlethal effects. Biochem J 1989;264:1–14.
27 Kojima S, Tsuchida M, Matsuyama T: Myelodysplasia and leukemia after treatment of aplastic anemia with G-CSF [letter]. N Engl J Med 1992;326:1294–1295.
28 Imashuku S, Hibi S, Kataoka-Morimoto Y, Yoshihara T, Ikushima S, Morioka Y, Todo S: Myelodysplasia and acute myeloid leukaemia in cases of aplastic anaemia and congenital neutropenia following G-CSF administration. Br J Haematol 1995;89:188–190.
29 Betticher DC, Huxol H, Müller R, Speck B, Nissen C: Colony growth in cultures from bone marrow and peripheral blood after curative treatment for leukemia and severe aplastic anemia. Exp Hematol 1993;21:1517–1521.
30 Rosti V, Tremml G, Soares V, Pandolfi PP, Luzzatto L, Bessler M: Murine embryonic stem cells without pig-a gene activity are competent for hematopoiesis with the PNH phenotype but not for clonal expansion [see comments]. J Clin Invest 1997; 100:1028–1036.
31 Brodsky RA, Vala MS, Barber JP, Medof ME, Jones RJ: Resistance to apoptosis caused by PIG-A gene mutations in paroxysmal nocturnal hemoglobinuria. Proc Natl Acad Sci USA 1997;94:8756–8760.
32 De Lord C, Tooze JA, Saso R, Marsh JC, Gordon-Smith EC: Deficiency of glycosylphosphatidyl inositol-anchored proteins in patients with aplastic anaemia does not affect response to immunosuppressive therapy. Br J Haematol 1998;101:90–93.
33 Iwamoto N, Kawaguchi T, Horikawa K, Nagakura S, Kagimoto T, Suda T, Takatsuki K, Nakakuma H: Preferential hematopoiesis by paroxysmal nocturnal hemoglobinuria clone engrafted in SCID mice. Blood 1996;87:4944–4948.

Acta Haematologica

Acta Haematol 2000;103:41–48

# Paroxysmal Nocturnal Haemoglobinuria: A Replacement of Haematopoietic Tissue?

Hubert Schrezenmeier[a] Anette Hildebrand[b] Markus Rojewski[a]
Hans Häcker[b] Hermann Heimpel[b] Aruna Raghavachar[b]

[a]Free University of Berlin, University Hospital Benjamin Franklin, Medical Clinic III, Berlin,
[b]University of Ulm, Department of Medicine III, Ulm, Germany

**Key Words**

Aplastic anaemia · Glycosylphosphatidyl-inositol anchor · Paroxysmal nocturnal haemoglobinuria · Pathophysiology · PIG-A gene

**Abstract**

Acquired somatic mutations of the PIG-A gene lead to deficient expression of glycosyl-phosphatidyl-inositol-anchored proteins (GPI-AP) by haematopoietic cells and play a causative role in the pathogenesis of paroxysmal nocturnal haemoglobinuria (PNH). However, PIG-A mutations do not explain how the defective PNH clone can expand. It was hypothesized that a selection process conferring a relative advantage to the GPI-AP-deficient population is required. Since GPI-AP-deficient cells are also detectable in a substantial proportion of patients with otherwise typical aplastic anaemia (AA), the mechanisms inducing bone marrow failure might selectively spare the GPI-deficient cells. In order to examine the growth characteristics of GPI-AP-deficient cells in more detail, we performed repeated analyses of GPI-AP expression on peripheral blood cells in 41 patients with AA. We observed four patterns of the course of GPI-AP-deficient populations: (1) 13 patients showed normal expression of GPI-AP in the first analysis and in at least two follow-up studies at a median time of 709 days after the first analysis. (2) Secondary evolution of a GPI-AP-deficient population was a rare event. Only 4 patients with initially normal GPI-AP expression developed a GPI-AP-deficient population during follow up after immunosuppressive treatment. (3) Persistence of GPI-AP-deficient cells was observed in 16 patients during a median follow-up time of 774 days. However, in some patients, the size of the GPI-AP-deficient population increased substantially. (4) Disappearance of a GPI-AP-deficient population was observed in 8 patients. The time course of GPI-AP expression in relation to the treatment suggests that therapeutic interventions might modulate the ratio of normal versus GPI-AP-deficient haematopoiesis. Overall, these data argue against an 'absolute growth advantage' of GPI-AP-deficient cells. Our data are consistent with the hypothesis that haematopoietic failure caused by damage to normal haematopoiesis allows the outgrowth of a GPI-AP-deficient population. Thus, in at least some patients GPI-AP-deficient cells might pre-exist at a very low percentage and replace haematopoiesis after an insult to the normal cells.



KARGER

Fax +41 61 306 12 34
E-Mail karger@karger.ch
www.karger.com


0001–5792/00/1031–0041$17.50/0

Accessible online at:
www.karger.com/journals/aha

H. Schrezenmeier, MD
Free University of Berlin, University Hospital Benjamin Franklin
Medical Clinic III, Hindenburgdamm 30
D–12200 Berlin (Germany)
Tel./Fax +49 30 8445 4551/4552, E-Mail schrezenmeier@ukbf.fu-berlin.de

## Introduction

Bruno Speck's group was interested in the clinical association between aplastic anaemia (AA) and paroxysmal nocturnal haemoglobinuria (PNH) long before the elucidation of the genetic basis of PNH [1]. They reported on a 25% actuarial risk of developing PNH at 15 years after immunosuppressive treatment of AA [1, 2]. The pathophysiological basis for this clinical observation has remained unclear for a long time. Over the past several years much progress has been accomplished in our understanding of the pathophysiology of PNH. It was demonstrated that acquired somatic mutations of the PIG-A gene resulting in the deficiency of glycosyl-phosphatidyl-inositol-anchored proteins (GPI-AP) are the molecular basis of PNH [3, 4]. GPI-AP-deficient cells are also present in a substantial proportion of patients with AA [5–10]. Consistent with these findings Bruno Speck's group demonstrated that the majority of patients with severe AA (SAA) transiently harbour complement-sensitive precursor cells in the bone marrow [11].

It is, however, not clear why a somatic mutation occurring in the PIG-A gene of a haematopoietic stem cell leads to a preferential expansion of the GPI-AP-deficient clone in PNH and the AA/PNH syndrome. Essentially there are two possibilities:

(1) the mutated cell might have a growth advantage over normal stem cells. If this is the case, the PIG-A mutation will cause a clonal dominance. However, so far there is no evidence for a proliferative advantage or a survival advantage of the mutated population [3,4, 12, 13].

(2) Alternatively, the PIG-A mutation does not change the growth characteristics of the affected cell. Impairment of the normal haemopoiesis by mechanisms which spare the GPI-AP-deficient clone might confer a relative growth advantage to the mutated clone [4, 12]. As a result, normal haematopoiesis will decrease while the size of the mutated clone will increase. Some of GPI-AP are important for adhesion and activation of lymphocytes and therefore GPI-AP-deficient cells might *escape* from an immune attack against haemopoietic cells due to the absence of a recognition site for cytotoxic lymphocytes [14]. This would mean that PNH cells are a 'replacement haematopoietic tissue' that might rescue patients from aplasia.

Here we present further evidence to support the hypothesis of a specific selection of GPI-AP-deficient cells. We have performed serial analyses of GPI-AP expression in 41 AA patients on granulocytes, monocytes, lymphocytes, erythrocytes and reticulocytes by flow cytometry. This longitudinal study demonstrates that the course of GPI-AP deficient populations is very heterogeneous. Besides the appearance of newly developed GPI-AP-deficient populations, persistence, expansion or disappearance of GPI-AP-deficient populations was observed.

## Patients and Methods

*Patients*

A total of 41 patients with AA were studied. This includes 32 patients whose initial GPI-AP state has been published previously [5]. In 25 patients, the first GPI-AP analysis was performed at diagnosis or at relapse, in 16 patients the initial analysis was performed during follow up after immunosuppressive treatment (IST). The criterion for inclusion in this analysis was the availability of at least two GPI-AP assessments with a minimum interval of 3 months. The median number of immunophenotypic investigations was 5 per patient (range 2–11).

The diagnosis of AA was established according to accepted criteria [15]. The severity of AA was recorded according to published criteria [15, 16]. Fourteen patients had non-severe AA, 21 SAA, and 6 very severe AA. All patients had IST. Twenty-eight patients received antilymphocyte globulin (ALG; Lymphoglobulin Mérieux) with cyclosporin A (CyA) and methylprednisolone (MP), one patient each received ALG + CyA + MP + interleukin-3 (Behring; Marburg, Germany) or ALG + CyA + MP + granulocyte colony-stimulating factor (Filgrastim; Amgen, Munich, Germany) and 1 patient was treated with ALG + MP. Ten patients were treated with CyA alone. Details on the treatment protocols have been published previously [5, 15, 17].

*Immunofluorescence*

Immunophenotyping was performed as previously described [5]. We analysed the expression of CD16, CD55 and CD66b on granulocytes, of CD14, CD48 and CD55 on monocytes, CD48, CD52 and CD59 on lymphocytes, and CD55, CD58 and CD59 on reticulocytes and erythrocytes. For analysis of reticulocytes 1 ml of phosphate-buffered saline with 0.1% (wt/vol) bovine serum albumin and 2 μl of an EDTA-anticoagulated venous blood sample were incubated with 1 ml of thiazol orange solution (Retic-count; Becton Dickinson, Heidelberg, Germany) for 20 min at room temperature. Staining of the reticulocytes by the RNA dye thiazol orange allowed for a separate analysis of erythrocytes and reticulocytes.

The limits for a significant GPI-AP-deficient population were as previously published [5]: 10.1% CD55-negative erythrocytes, 4.1% CD48-negative lymphocytes, 9.7% CD14- negative and 4.5% CD48-negative monocytes, 4.4% CD16-negative and 2.5% CD66b-negative granulocytes. In order to be considered as a significant GPI-AP deficient population, a GPI-AP-negative population in AA patients had to exceed these limits.

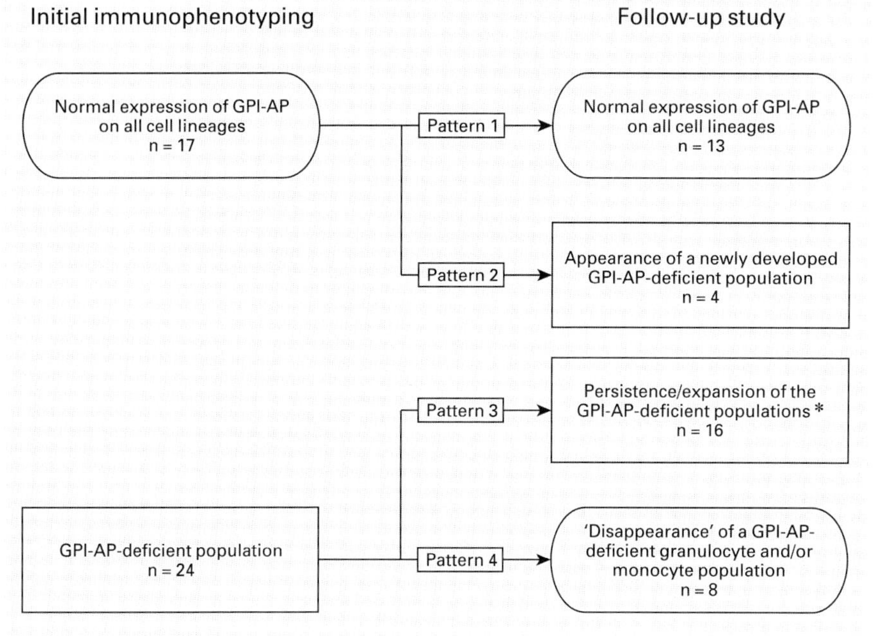


**Fig. 1.** Summary of the results of repeated analysis of GPI-AP expression on peripheral blood cells in 41 patients with AA.

## Results

We performed repeated assessments of GPI-AP expression on granulocytes, monocytes, lymphocytes, erythrocytes and reticulocytes in 41 patients with AA. The median interval between the first and the latest immunophenotypic analysis of GPI-AP expression was 889 days. Results are summarised in figure 1. The longitudinal studies revealed four different patterns of GPI-AP expression during the follow-up of AA patients (fig. 1):

1 normal expression of GPI-AP during the entire investigation period (pattern 1);
2 appearance of a newly developed GPI-AP-deficient population during follow up (pattern 2);
3 persistence or expansion of a GPI-AP-deficient population (pattern 3), and
4 'Disappearance' of a GPI-AP-deficient population (pattern 4).

*Pattern 1*

Seventeen patients had normal expression of GPI-AP at first analysis. In 13 of these patients, expression of GPI-AP on all cell lineages was also normal in at least two follow-up studies which were performed at a median time of 709 days after the first analysis.

*Pattern 2*

Four patients with initially normal expression of GPI-AP developed a GPI-AP-deficient population during follow-up. Two patients developed a CD16-, CD66b- and CD55-negative granulocyte population and a CD14-, CD48- and CD55-negative monocyte population 405 and 469 days after the first analysis. In two other patients a CD14-, CD48- and CD55-negative monocyte population and a CD48-, CD52- and CD59-negative lymphocyte population appeared 154 and 404 days after diagnosis. Three of these patients still had bone marrow aplasia with pancytopenia at the time of appearance of the GPI-AP-deficient population. Only 1 patient developed the newly appearing GPI-AP-deficient population in clinical remission after IST.

*Pattern 3*

Persistence of a GPI-AP-deficient population was observed in 16 patients. At least two follow-up studies were performed in each patient after a median follow-up of 774 days since the first immunophenotyping of GPI-AP. The proportion of GPI-AP-deficient granulocytes in these 16 patients is shown in figure 2. The relative proportion of GPI-AP-deficient cells varied considerably over time. In some patients, the GPI-AP-deficient population increased gradually during follow-up.

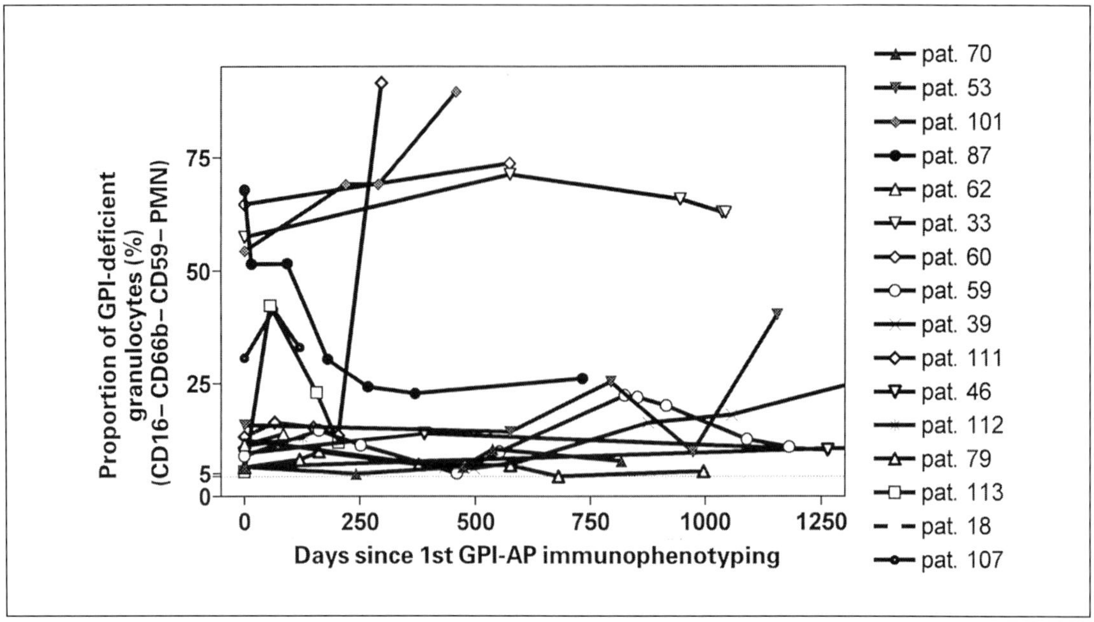


**Fig. 2.** Persistence of GPI-AP-deficient cells during long-term follow-up after IST of AA. The graph shows the percentage of CD16-, CD66b and CD55-negative granulocytes in 16 patients with AA (median follow-up after first immunophenotyping of GPI-AP: 774 days).

The time course of GPI-AP-deficient cells in patient No. 101 exemplifies the expansion of the GPI-AP-deficient clone (fig. 3). When the patient presented with a relapse of AA 8.2 years after diagnosis, a small but significant proportion of monocytes and granulocytes were GPI-AP-deficient. During treatment with CsA, the patient achieved a partial response. Both the relative proportion and the absolute count of GPI-AP-deficient red cells, monocytes and granulocytes increased continuously (fig. 3). Thus, in this case, the haematopoietic recovery was due to an expansion of the GPI-AP deficient clone during CsA treatment.

In 5 of the patients with persistence of a GPI-AP-deficient granulocyte and monocyte population, a GPI-AP-deficient lymphocyte population that was not detectable at first analysis appeared during follow-up. The size of the GPI-AP-deficient lymphocyte population was small in these patients. The median proportion of CD48-negative lymphocytes was 7.4%.

*Pattern 4*

Disappearance of a GPI-AP-deficient population was observed in 8 patients who presented with a significant GPI-AP-deficient granulocyte and monocyte population at diagnosis (n = 6) or at relapse (n = 2) (fig. 4a). The median time between the initial immunophenotyping and the disappearance of the GPI-AP-deficient population in these 8 patients was 358 days. The median proportion of CD16-, CD55- and CD66b-negative granulocytes was 15.9% at the initial investigation, when the patients presented with cytopenia and declined to 0.7% during follow-up. As an example the immunophenotyping of CD16, CD55 and CD66b expression on granulocytes of 2 patients at diagnosis and after 533 and 553 days is shown in figure 4b.

In all but 1 patient, the decline of the GPI-AP-deficient population was associated with haematopoietic recovery. However, in 5 of these patients, the haematological improvement was delayed and in 2 patients it was obtained only after sequential courses of IST.

## Discussion

It has been demonstrated that acquired somatic mutations of the PIG-A gene in an early haematopoietic progenitor cell are the genetic basis of PNH [18–31]. It has been shown by several groups that GPI-AP-deficient cells are also present in a substantial proportion of patients with AA [5, 6, 8, 9]. Investigations on the evolution of the

GPI-AP-deficient cells and their impact on the course of AA might provide insights into the mechanism regulating their growth. Therefore we have performed repeated assessments of GPI-AP expression in AA patients. The course of the GPI-AP-deficient populations was heterogeneous. In 16 of 24 AA patients in whom we could detect a GPI-AP-deficient population at first analysis, we observed persistence or even expansion of the GPI-AP-deficient population. One might speculate that in these cases the mechanism (e.g. immune attack) sparing the GPI-AP-deficient clone has persisted. In some patients, the selection mechanism might be modulated by therapeutic interventions (e.g CsA) as suggested by the course of the GPI-AP-deficient population in patient No. 101 and in a case reported by Nakao et al. [32]. These are further examples emphasizing that in occasional patients the expansion of a GPI-AP-deficient population might rescue the patient from aplasia [33]. However, in most of our patients CsA treatment did not lead to an expansion of the GPI-AP-deficient population, nor was a CsA-induced expansion of the PNH clone seen in any of the patients described in a recent report by van Kamp et al. [34].

In some AA patients, GPI-AP-deficient populations disappeared. This is the first demonstration of disappearance of a GPI-AP-deficient granulocyte or monocyte population in *typical AA* along with haematopoietic recovery. Disappearance of a PNH clone was observed in some PNH patients with spontaneous remissions [35–37] and in a patient with the AA/PNH syndrome after complete response to ALG [38]. It is not clear whether the GPI-AP-deficient clone is completely eliminated in patients with 'disappearance' of a GPI-AP-deficient population or whether the clone is reduced to an undetectable size. Persistence of GPI-AP-deficient T lymphocytes was demonstrated in long-term clinical remission of PNH [36, 39]. In patients in whom the GPI-AP-deficient granulocyte population disappeared, we could not detect any significant number of GPI-AP-deficient lymphocytes.

In a SCID mouse model preferential engraftment of PNH clones was observed as compared to normal haematopoiesis [40]. This was attributed to a growth advantage of the PNH clone brought about by an endogenous growth abnormality of the PNH clone [40]. In contrast, in chimaeric mice generated by targeted disruption of the murine homologue of the PIG-A gene, the proportion of GPI-AP-deficient cells was low and remained stable for 10 months after birth and there was no apparent growth advantage of the PIG-A mutated cells [41, 42]. The course of GPI-AP-deficient cells in group 3 very much resembles the course of the GPI-AP-deficient population in the chi-

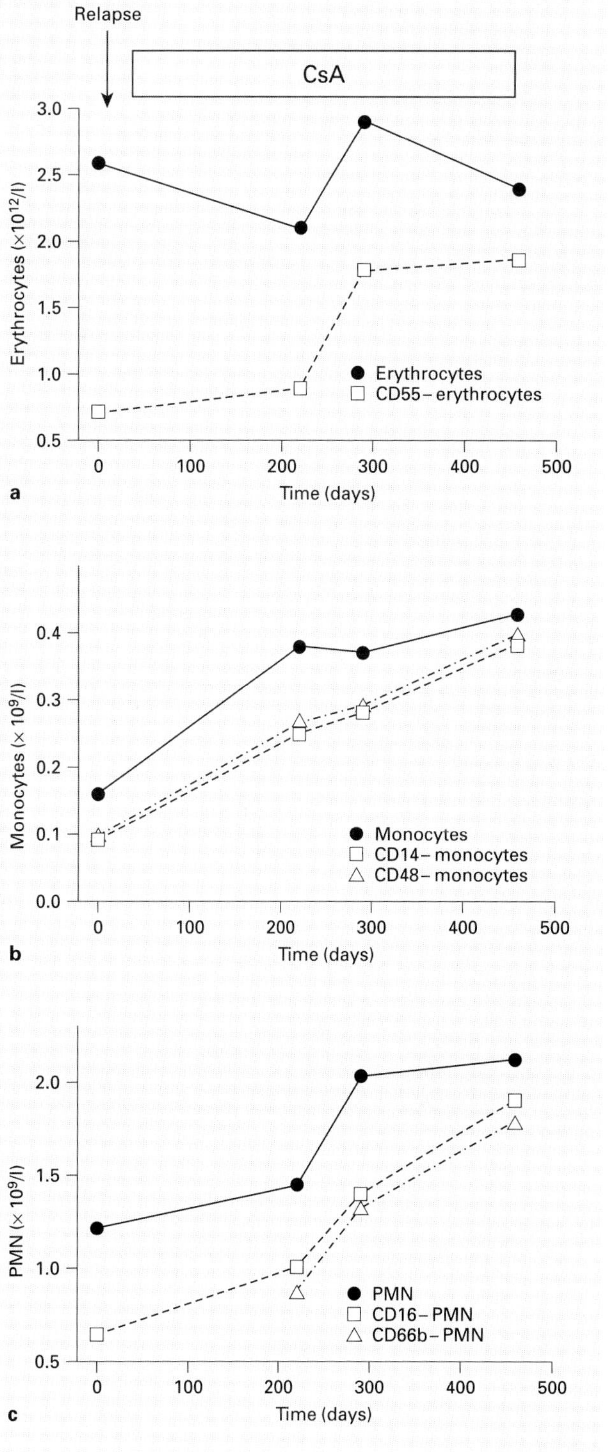


**Fig. 3.** Expansion of GPI-AP-deficient populations. Time course of red cells, monocytes and granulocytes (closed symbols) of patient No. 1 during CsA treatment after diagnosis of a relapse. The open symbols indicate the absolute count of CD55-negative red cells (**a**), CD48- and CD14-negative monocytes (**b**) and CD16- and CD66b-negative granulocytes (**c**).

Fig. 4. Disappearance of GPI-AP-deficient cells. **a** The graph shows the percentage of CD16- , CD66b and CD55-negative granulocytes at the time of diagnosis of the PNH cells and at follow-up in 8 patients with AA. **b**, **c** Flow-cytometric analysis of CD16, CD66b and CD55 on granulocytes of patient No. 38 (**b**) and patient No. 66 (**c**) at diagnosis and 553 and 533 days later. Both patients had achieved a response to treatment at the time of the follow-up analysis. --- = Irrelevant control antibody as negative control; black areas = specific anti-GPI-AP antibody.

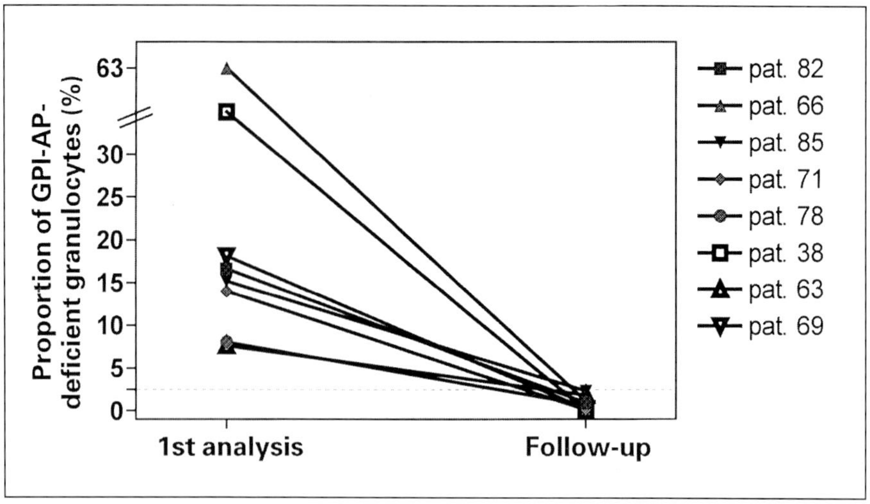

a

naeric mouse models with targeted disruption of the PIG-A gene [41, 42].

In keeping with other results, the disappearance of a GPI-AP-deficient population in about one third of AA patients with a GPI-AP-deficient population argues against a general survival and growth advantage of PNH clones over normal cells. As measured in both primary colony cultures and long-term marrow culture assays, no intrinsic growth advantage of GPI-AP-deficient progenitor cells could be demonstrated [43]. These observations show that a PIG-A mutation alone does not immediately cause a clonal dominance of GPI-AP-deficient cells. If a sufficient number of normal haematopoietic cells is present, GPI-AP-deficient cells are 'diluted' in normal cells and no 'replacement tissue' is necessary.

The results of our longitudinal study support the hypothesis that haematopoietic failure caused by damage to the normal cells might confer a relative advantage to the GPI-AP-deficient population. The persistence or expansion of the GPI-AP-deficient clone depends on a reversible selection mechanism which might be modulated by immunosuppressive treatment. The nature of a selection mechanism which operates in PNH or AA and leads to a selective expansion of GPI-AP-deficient cells is not yet clear. We and others demonstrated that selection of GPI-AP-deficient cells by an immunological mechanism is possible. In vivo application of the cytotoxic Campath-1H antibody which is directed against the GPI-AP CD52 led to a reversible emergence of GPI-AP-deficient lymphocytes and monocytes [44, 45]. The association of low endogenous IL-2 release with progression of AA to PNH points at the potential importance of immunological mechanisms for the selection of PNH cells in vivo [11].

In summary, our data are in keeping with the hypothesis that the occurrence of a GPI-AP-deficient clone requires at least two independent pathogenetic steps: a PIG-A gene mutation is a prerequisite. However, a PIG-A mutation does not inevitably lead to an expansion of a clonal GPI-AP-deficient population. In addition, a selection process is required which causes a preferential expansion of the GPI-AP-deficient clone. Insight into the nature of these selection processes can open new concepts for the treatment of PNH and the AA/PNH syndrome.

The different growth properties of GPI-AP-deficient cells in AA patients might reflect the heterogeneity of PIG-A mutations. One might speculate that some PIG-A mutations confer a growth advantage (or disadvantage) to the mutated cells whereas other PIG-A mutations do not affect growth and survival of the affected cells.


## Acknowledgments

We thank A. Szmaragowska, A. Fischer, C. Schöpflin and I. Lüthje for skilful technical assistance. This work was supported by the Deutsche Forschungsgemeinschaft (SFB 322) and the European Commission (BIOMED 2, BMH4-CT96-1031).

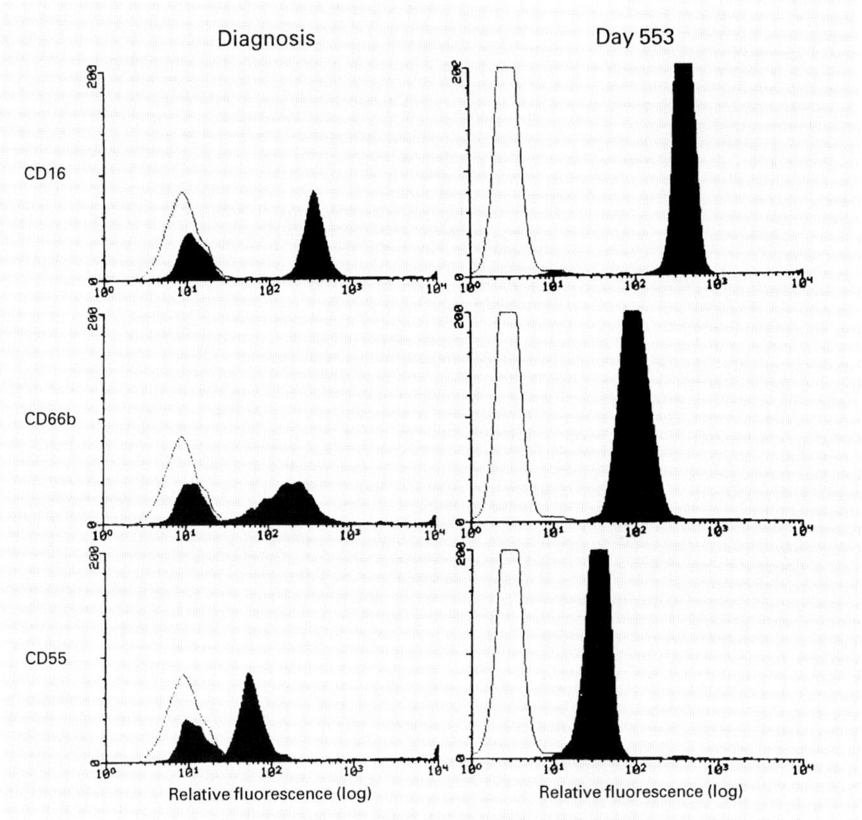
Diagnosis
Day 553
CD16
CD66b
CD55
Relative fluorescence (log)
Relative fluorescence (log)

**b**

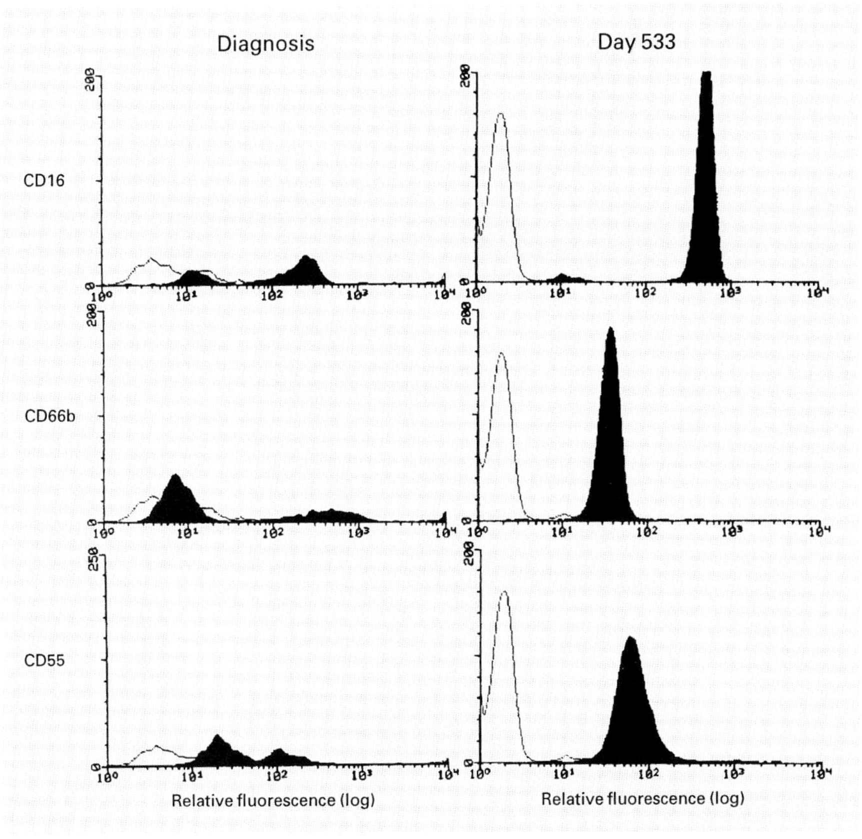
Diagnosis
Day 533
CD16
CD66b
CD55
Relative fluorescence (log)
Relative fluorescence (log)

**c**

## References


1 Tichelli A, Gratwohl A, Wursch A, et al: Late haematological complications in severe aplastic anaemia. Br J Haematol 1988;69:413–418.
2 Tichelli A, Gratwohl A, Nissen C, et al: Late clonal complications in severe aplastic anemia. Leuk Lymphoma 1994;12:167–175.
3 Rosse WF, Ware RE: The molecular basis of paroxysmal nocturnal hemoglobinuria. Blood 1995;86:3277–3286.
4 Luzzatto L, Bessler M: The dual pathogenesis of paroxysmal nocturnal hemoglobinuria. Curr Opin Hematol 1996;3:101–110.
5 Schrezenmeier H, Hertenstein B, Wagner B, et al: A pathogenetic link between aplastic anemia and paroxysmal nocturnal hemoglobinuria is suggested by a high frequency of aplastic anemia patients with a deficiency of phosphatidylinositol glycan anchored proteins. Exp Hematol 1995;23:81–87.
6 Dunn DE, Tanawattanacharoen P, Boccuni P, et al: Paroxysmal nocturnal hemoglobinuria cells in patients with bone marrow failure syndromes (see comments). Ann Intern Med 1999; 131:401–408.
7 Fores R, Alcocer M, Diez Martin JL, et al: Flow cytometric analysis of decay-accelerating factor (CD55) on neutrophils from aplastic anaemia patients. Br J Haematol 1995;90:728–730.
8 Griscelli Bennaceur A, Gluckman E, Scrobohaci ML, et al: Aplastic anemia and paroxysmal nocturnal hemoglobinuria: Search for a pathogenetic link. Blood 1995;85:1354–1363.
9 Schubert J, Vogt HG, Zielinska Skowronek M, et al: Development of the glycosylphosphatitylinositol-anchoring defect characteristic for paroxysmal nocturnal hemoglobinuria in patients with aplastic anemia. Blood 1994;83:2323–2328.
10 Tooze JA, Saso R, Marsh JC, et al: The novel monoclonal antibody By114 helps detect the early emergence of a paroxysmal nocturnal hemoglobinuria clone in aplastic anemia. Exp Hematol 1995;23:1484–1491.
11 Nissen C, Tichelli A, Gratwohl A, et al: High incidence of transiently appearing complement-sensitive bone marrow precursor cells in patients with severe aplastic anemia: A possible role of high endogenous IL-2 in their suppression. Acta Haematol 1999;101:165–172.
12 Rotoli B, Luzzatto L: Paroxysmal nocturnal haemoglobinuria. Baillières Clin Haematol 1989;2:113–138.
13 Rotoli B, Bessler M, Alfinito F, et al: Membrane proteins in paroxysmal nocturnal haemoglobinuria. Blood Rev 1993;7:75–86.
14 Young NS: The problem of clonality in aplastic anemia: Dr Dameshek's riddle, restated. Blood 1992;79:1385–1392.
15 Frickhofen N, Kaltwasser JP, Schrezenmeier H, et al: Treatment of aplastic anemia with antilymphocyte globulin and methylprednisolone with or without cyclosporine. N Engl J Med 1991;324:1297–1304.
16 Bacigalupo A, Hows J, Gluckman E, et al: Bone marrow transplantation (BMT) versus immunosuppression for the treatment of severe aplastic anaemia (SAA): A report of the EBMT SAA working party. Br J Haematol 1988;70: 177–182.
17 Raghavachar A, Ganser A, Freund M, et al: Long-term interleukin-3 and intensive immunosuppression in the treatment of aplastic anemia. Cytokines Mol Ther 1996;215–223.
18 Bessler M, Mason PJ, Hillmen P, et al: Paroxysmal nocturnal haemoglobinuria (PNH) is caused by somatic mutations in the PIG-A gene. EMBO J 1994;13:110–117.
19 Bessler M, Mason P, Hillmen P, et al: Somatic mutations and cellular selection in paroxysmal nocturnal haemoglobinuria. Lancet 1994;343: 951–953.
20 Bessler M, Mason PJ, Hillmen P, et al: Mutations in the PIG-A gene causing partial deficiency of GPI-linked surface proteins (PNH II) in patients with paroxysmal nocturnal haemoglobinuria. Br J Haematol 1994;87:863–866.
21 Miyata T, Takeda J, Iida Y, et al: The cloning of PIG-A, a component in the early step of GPI-anchor biosynthesis. Science 1993;259: 1318–1320.
22 Ostendorf T, Nischan C, Schubert J, et al: Heterogeneous PIG-A mutations in different cell lineages in paroxysmal nocturnal hemoglobinuria heterogeneous PIG-A mutations in different cell lineages in paroxysmal nocturnal hemoglobinuria. Blood 1995;85:1640–1646.
23 Takeda J, Miyata T, Kawagoe K, et al: Deficiency of the GPI anchor caused by a somatic mutation of the PIG-A gene in paroxysmal nocturnal hemoglobinuria deficiency of the GPI anchor caused by a somatic mutation of the PIG-A gene in paroxysmal nocturnal hemoglobinuria. Cell 1993;73:703–711.
24 Ware RE, Rosse WF, Howard TA: Mutations within the Piga gene in patients with paroxysmal nocturnal hemoglobinuria. Blood 1994;83: 2418–2422.
25 Yamada N, Miyata T, Maeda K, et al: Somatic mutations of the PIG-A gene found in Japanese patients with paroxysmal nocturnal hemoglobinuria. Blood 1995;85:885–892.
26 Endo M, Ware RE, Vreeke TM, et al: Molecular basis of the heterogeneity of expression of glycosyl phosphatidylinositol anchored proteins in paroxysmal nocturnal hemoglobinuria. Blood 1996;87:2546–2557.
27 Lin LI, Liu CH, Chen YC, et al: PIG-A gene mutations in four Taiwanese patients with paroxysmal nocturnal haemoglobinuria following aplastic anaemia. Br J Haematol 1997;97:286–292.
28 Nafa K, Mason PJ, Hillmen P, et al: Mutations in the PIG-A gene causing paroxysmal nocturnal hemoglobinuria are mainly of the frameshift type. Blood 1995;86:4650–4655.
29 Nagarajan S, Brodsky RA, Young NS, et al: Genetic defects underlying paroxysmal nocturnal hemoglobinuria that arises out of aplastic anemia. Blood 1995;86:4656–4661.
30 Nishimura J, Inoue N, Wada H, et al: A patient with paroxysmal nocturnal hemoglobinuria bearing four independent PIG-A mutant clones. Blood 1997;89:3470–3476.
31 Savoia A, Ianzano L, Lunardi C, et al: Identification of three novel mutations in the PIG-A gene in paroxysmal nocturnal haemoglobinuria (PNH) patients. Hum Genet 1996;97:45–48.
32 Nakao S, Yamaguchi M, Takamatsu H, et al: Expansion of a paroxysmal nocturnal hemoglobinuria (PNH) clone after cyclosporine therapy for aplastic anemia/PNH syndrome (letter; comment). Blood 1992;80:2943–2944.
33 Hillmen P, Hows JM, Luzzatto L: Two distinct patterns of glycosylphosphatidylinositol (GPI) linked protein deficiency in the red cells of patients with paroxysmal nocturnal haemoglobinuria. Br J Haematol 1992;80:399–405.
34 van Kamp H, van Imhoff GW, de Wolf JT, et al: The effect of cyclosporine on haematological parameters in patients with paroxysmal nocturnal haemoglobinuria. Br J Haematol 1995; 89:79–82.
35 Dacie J: Paroxysmal nocturnal haemoglobinuria. Sangre 1980;25:890–895.
36 Hillmen P, Bessler M, Luzzatto L, et al: Long-term follow-up of 80 patients with PNH: 11 of 32 patients surviving 10 years achieve spontaneous remission (abstract). Blood 1993;82 (suppl 1):310a.
37 Hillmen P, Lewis SM, Bessler M, et al: Natural history of paroxysmal nocturnal hemoglobinuria. N Engl J Med 1995;333:1253–1258.
38 Kusminsky GD, Barazzutti L, Korin JD, et al: Complete response to antilymphocyte globulin in a case of aplastic anemia-paroxysmal nocturnal hemoglobinuria syndrome (letter). Am J Hematol 1988;29:123.
39 Nakakuma H, Nagakura S, Kawaguchi T, et al: Persistence of affected T lymphoctes in long-term clinical remission in paroxysmal nocturnal hemoglobinuria. Blood 1994;84:3925–3928.
40 Iwamoto N, Kawaguchi T, Horikawa K, et al: Preferential hematopoiesis by paroxysmal nocturnal hemoglobinuria clone engrafted in SCID mice. Blood 1996;87:4944–4948.
41 Kawagoe K, Kitamura D, Okabe M, et al: Glycosylphosphatidylinositol-anchor-deficient mice: Implications for clonal dominance of mutant cells in paroxysmal nocturnal hemoglobinuria. Blood 1996;87:3600–3606.
42 Keller P, Tremml G, Rosti V, et al: X inactivation and somatic cell selection rescue female mice carrying a Piga-null mutation. Proc Natl Acad Sci USA 1999;96:7479–7483.
43 Maciejewski JP, Sloand EM, Sato T, et al: Impaired hematopoiesis in paroxysmal nocturnal hemoglobinuria / aplastic anemia is not associated with a selective proliferative defect in the glycosylphosphatidylinositol-anchored protein-deficient clone. Blood 1997;89:1173–1181.
44 Brett SJ, Baxter G, Cooper H, et al: Emergence of CD52-, glycosylphosphatidylinositol-anchor-deficient lymphocytes in rheumatoid arthritis patients following Campath-1 treatment. Int Immunol 1996;8:325–334.
45 Hertenstein B, Wagner B, Bunjes D, et al: Emergence of CD52-, phosphatidylinositolglycan-anchor-deficient T lymphocytes after in vivo application of Campath-1H for refractory B-cell Non-Hodgkin Lymphoma Emergence of CD52-, phosphatidylinositolglycan-anchor-deficient T lymphocytes after in vivo application of Campath-1H for refractory B-cell non-Hodgkin lymphoma. Blood 1995;86:1487–1492.

Acta Hæmatologica

Acta Haematol 2000;103:49–54

# Cure from Severe Aplastic Anemia in vivo and Late Effects

Gérard Socié Eliane Gluckman

Service d'Hématologie-Greffe de Moelle, Hôpital Saint-Louis, Paris, France

**Key Words**
Aplastic anemia · Long-term survival · Secondary malignancies

**Abstract**
Recent progress in the treatment of aplastic anemia has dramatically changed the previously grim prognosis for these patients. Improvements in bone marrow transplantation and immunosuppression have increased the number of long-term survivors so that immediate survival is no longer the sole concern. Here, were review the major clinical studies and summarize recent analyses of late malignant and nonmalignant complications following treatment of aplastic anemia.



## Introduction

Recent progress in the treatment of aplastic anemia has dramatically changed the previously grim prognosis of these patients: today the 2-year survival is 60–90%. Improved results following bone marrow transplantation or immunosuppression increase the number of patients alive years after presentation, thus immediate survival is no longer the sole concern. Indeed, quality of life and late complications are becoming increasingly important. However, there are fundamental differences between the two major treatment modalities, resulting in their having specific effects on late morbidity and long-term survival.

Patients are likely to be cured of aplastic anemia by successful marrow transplantation. Late effects are caused by the treatment used to prepare the patient for transplantation and the extent of chronic graft-versus-host disease (GVHD) and its treatment rather than the underlying disease. In contrast, after immunosuppression, recovery often takes several months and the stigmata of the disease persist despite clinical remission. Although immunosuppression allows autologous reconstitution of hemopoiesis, it leaves the patient with a fragile bone marrow prone to the development of a clonal disorder, such as myelodysplastic syndrome (MDS) or paroxysmal nocturnal hemoglobinuria (PNH). The interrelationship between PNH and severe aplastic anemia is reviewed by Schrezenmeier [1] in this issue. We will briefly review the problem of MDS and leukemia, the development of solid tumors and the long-term outcome of patients who underwent allogeneic transplantation or who received immunosuppressive therapy.

## Secondary MDS or Leukemia

In 1998, two single-center studies described the evolution of acquired aplastic anemia to MDS or leukemia in patients treated with immunosuppression. In Leiden, 5 of 35 patients with aplastic anemia surviving for 2 or more

KARGER
Fax +41 61 306 12 34
E-Mail karger@karger.ch
www.karger.com


0001–5792/00/1031–0049$17.50/0

Accessible online at:
www.karger.com/journals/aha

G. Socié, MD, PhD
Service d'Hématologie Greffe de Moelle, Hôpital Saint Louis
1, avenue Claude-Vellefaux
F–75475 Paris Cedex 10 (France)
Tel. +33 1 42 49 98 24, Fax +33 1 42 41 14 70

years developed MDS [2]. All 5 patients had a normal karyotype at the time of first diagnosis: 3 of them were treated with antilymphocyte globulin (ALG) corticosteroids and androgens, and 2 received corticosteroids and androgens and were splenectomized. A pattern of evolution could be identified in patients with secondary hematological malignancy. The aplastic marrow first showed an improvement in hemopoiesis and subsequently developed dysplastic features in one or more cell lines, predominantly dyserythropoiesis. Refractory anemia evolved into chronic myelomonocytic leukemia in 2 patients, and refractory anemia with an excess of blasts in 1 patient. Three patients had an abnormal karyotype with monosomy 7 at the time of the secondary MDS. Overall, 10% of all patients surviving for 2 years eventually developed a leukemic disorder.

Similarly, the Basel group reviewed late hematological disorders in 137 patients with aplastic anemia [3]. One hundred and three patients were treated with ALG and 34 with bone marrow transplantation. Twenty of the 103 patients treated with immunosuppression showed a clonal evolution (8 MDS; 12 PNH; 1 MDS/PNH), but this did not occur in any of the patients treated with bone marrow transplantation. The risk of developing a hematological complication after immunosuppressive treatment was 57% at 8 years. In a subsequent follow-up study, it was found that cytogenetic analysis at diagnosis was normal in 13 patients who developed MDS/leukemia. At the time of transformation into malignant disease, patients presented a clonal abnormality on karyotype analysis: monosomy 6 was found in 2 patients, and 3 others had monosomy 7, deletion 7, deletion 14, or translocation t(8;21) respectively [4].

Long-term follow-up was evaluated in a large retrospective multicenter European Bone Marrow Transplantation (EBMT) group study including 468 aplastic anemia patients treated with ALG [5]. After immunosuppressive treatment of both severe and moderate aplastic anemia, the survival curve followed a biphasic pattern. The death rate was high in the first 2 years after treatment, but thereafter, mortality gradually declined. Of the 245 patients who survived for 2 years, 21 later died: 13 of hemorrhage or infection due to persistent pancytopenia, 4 of the consequences of PNH, and 4 of leukemia. Between the second and third years, pancytopenia due to aplastic anemia was still the major cause of death among long-term survivors; after the third year posttreatment, leukemia and MDS became the primary cause of death. Twelve patients developed MDS/leukemia at a median of 4.6 years after immunosuppression. The actuarial mortality of long-term survivors was 22% at 8 years, but so far no plateau has occurred. The 5-year actuarial probability of developing MDS was between 15 and 20%. In comparison to single-center studies [6, 7], the incidence of a clonal disease may have been underestimated, as these diagnoses are easily missed in the absence of symptoms without the appropriate and systematic blood and marrow tests.

To examine the incidence of hematological cancers and solid tumors in a large cohort of long-term survivors after treatment of aplastic anemia, the EBMT Severe Aplastic Anemia (SAA) Working Party studied the cases reported to the registry [8]. The study population consisted of 860 patients treated with immunosuppression and 748 patients who had received bone marrow transplants. The risk of malignancy was analyzed overall and according to treatment relative to the risk in the general population. Thirty-four of the 860 patients who underwent immunosuppressive treatment developed MDS or leukemia (19 DMS, 15 leukemia), as did 2 of the 748 patients who received bone marrow transplants. The risk factors for MDS or acute leukemia after immunosuppressive treatment included older age (relative risk or RR = 1.03), treatment in or after 1982, as compared with in or before 1981 (RR = 3.01), splenectomy (RR = 3.65), and multiple courses of immunosuppression (RR = 2.26). The addition of androgens to the immunosuppressive treatment was associated with a lower risk of malignancy (RR = 0.28). This study definitively proved the increased risk of developing MDS and leukemia after immunosuppressive treatment.

Recent findings have suggested that administration of G-CSF was associated with the development of MDS/leukemia. These data come mainly from Japan [9, 10]. In a study of 167 children with aplastic anemia, 11 of 50 patients treated with G-CSF and cyclosporin developed MDS/leukemia [9]. Of the group of children treated with G-CSF or cyclosporin alone, none had this complication. The 7-year probability of developing MDS/leukemia was 47 ± 17% for patients treated with growth factors as compared to 16 ± 6% for the whole cohort. Furthermore, patients treated for longer periods or with a higher cumulative growth factor doses seemed to be at an increased risk. Eight of the 11 late clonal disorders developed within 36 months, much earlier than is usually reported. These results were not corroborated in the prospective pilot study from Europe that included 40 patients treated with G-CSF, ALG and cyclosporin [11]. In a recent up-date, the frequency of MDS/leukemia in the 100 patients treated with this combination had not increased [A. Bacigalupo, pers. commun.]. The debate continues as to whether G-CSF is involved in the development of abnormal cytogenetics, the expension of premalignant clones and in leukemic transformations in immunosuppressed patients. Further studies are needed to identify risk factors for developing MDS/leukemia in patients with aplastic anemia with new combinations of immunosuppressive treatment.

Clinical observations indicate that there is a relationship between aplastic anemia and leukemic disorders, and all centers which have routinely tested patients at regular intervals report an actuarial risk of MDS and leukemia of between 10 and 20% at 10 years. The higher frequency of clonal complications observed since the mid-1980s can be accounted for by two factors: first, the improved survival of patients treated with immunosuppression, who otherwise would have died from pancytopenia, and, second, the systematic search for MDS in long-term patients. Indeed, studies that observed patients for only a short follow-up period failed to demonstrate an increased risk of leukemia [12, 13].

In contrast, hematological clonal complications are not usually observed after successful bone marrow transplantation. In a Seattle study, none of 168 transplanted patients developed leukemia. Twenty of 227 patients who received immunosuppressive treatment at the same institution developed secondary MDS or leukemia ($p = 0.001$) [7]. In fact, leukemia after successful bone marrow transplantation is extremely rare. A previous study from Seattle showed that only 1 of over 400 patients transplanted for aplastic anemia, whose conditioning regimen included cyclophosphamide, developed acute leukemia in host cells, 7 months after the transplantation [14]. Cytogenetics and polymerase chain reaction of microsatellite sequences proved that, in 2 instances, donor cell leukemia developed after transplantation [15].

It is not clear whether aplastic anemia is a preleukemic disorder. Clinical and biological evidence currently support the existence of a clear link between aplastic anemia and leukemia. Therefore, the high frequency of secondary leukemia is likely inherent in the disease rather than secondary to the immunosuppressive treatments.

Cytogenetic analysis demonstrates clonal changes before overt MDS or leukemia develops. In an early survey from Seattle, an abnormal karyotype was detected in 7 of 183 (4%) patients with otherwise morphologically typical aplastic anemia, 3 of the 7 patients were treated with immunosuppression and 2 developed late MDS or leukemia. Among the 169 patients with typical aplastic anemia without cytogenetic anomalies, 5 (3%) subsequently presented a leukemic transformation [16]. In an Italian study, bone marrow cells from 69 patients with acquired aplastic anemia were analyzed cytogenetically at diagnosis and after immunosuppressive treatment [17]: 51 patients (74%) were normal and remained so, but 18 patients (26%) had at least one abnormal karyotype. Remarkably, three patterns of evolution were observed. In 7 patients the anomaly was acquired after treatment, in 3 patients it was present at diagnosis and persisted during evolution, and in 8 patients it represented a transient posttreatment abnormality.

The EBMT SAA Working Party retrospectively evaluated cytogenetic anomalies in patients with aplastic anemia treated with immunosuppression between 1974 and 1994. One hundred and seventy evaluable karyotypes from six European centers were reported for analyses. One hundred and forty-six patients had normal karyotypes and 1 patient had a somatic chromosomal defect. In 23 cases (12%) chromosomal aberration in hemopoietic cells could be demonstrated. The anomaly was clonal in 19 of the 23 (11%) cases.

In Japan, monosomy 7 was the main chromosomal anomaly reported to occur in children treated with G-CSF and cyclosporin. Out of 11 children who developed MDS/leukemia, 8 had monosomy 7, 2 monosomy 7 together with monosomy 21, and 1 had a monosomy 21 clone [18].

All these reports show that a single clonal chromosomal defect in hemopoietic cells is not infrequent in aplastic anemia at presentation. Trisomy 8 and monosomy 7 are the most usual aberrations. However, cytogenetic analysis of empty marrow may be technically difficult, and classic karyotyping upon diagnosis of severe aplastic anemia is often not possible because of a lack of metaphases. Interphase fluorescent in situ hybridization (FISH) may detect anomalies such as trisomies and monosomies, even in marrow from patients in whom no metaphases are found.

## New Solid Cancers

Among late effects occurring after allogeneic bone marrow transplantation, solid cancers cause particular concern, and their occurrence needs to be quantified in large populations.

### *New Solid Cancers after Allogeneic Bone Marrow Transplantation*

Since the conditioning regimen for patients with aplastic anemia is different from that for other patients requiring allogeneic bone marrow transplants, the risk of developing solid tumors had to be determined specifically for this cohort. In a study from St. Louis Hospital, Paris, 147 patients with aplastic anemia (107 with acquired aplastic anemia; 40 with Fanconi's anemia) transplanted between 1980 and 1989 were evaluated for new cancers. The conditioning regimen included cyclophosphamide and thoracoabdominal irradiation. Four of the 147 patients developed a solid malignant tumor, all within the radiation field, and the 8-year cumulative incidence rate was 22% [19]. In Seattle, 5 of 330 transplanted patients with aplastic anemia developed secondary cancers: 318 patients had acquired aplastic anemia and 12 patients Fanconi's anemia [20]. The cumulative incidence of secondary cancers was 1.4% at 10 years, and 4.2% at 15 years. This report illustrates a remarkably lower risk of secondary tumors as compared to the results from Paris, a difference that may be accounted for by the exclusion of irradiation from the conditioning regimen and the lower proportion of Fanconi's anemia patients in the Seattle group compared to Paris (4% versus 27% in the French cohort). The influence of graft-versus-host disease and its treatment could not be determined.

The EBMT SAA Working Party examined the incidence of solid tumors in long-term survivors after treatment of aplastic anemia [8]. The risk of cancer was analyzed overall and according to treatment relative to the risk in the general population. Seven tumors occurred in the 748 patients who received bone marrow transplants. The overall relative risk of cancer after transplantation, as compared with that in the general European population, was 6.7 ($p < 0.001$). The 10-year cumulative incidence rate of cancer was 3.1%. Risk factors for solid cancers after bone marrow transplantation were found to be age (RR = 1.11 per year) and the use of irradiation as a conditioning regimen before transplantation (RR = 9.56); such tumors occurred only in male patients.

As the risk factors for developing new malignancies after marrow transplantation have not been fully defined, a retrospective joint Seattle and Paris analysis was performed on data from 700 patients treated with allogeneic bone marrow transplantation [21]. Twenty-three patients developed a malignancy 1.4–221 months after transplantation, with an actuarial probability of 14% at 20 years. Five cases were lymphoid malignancies occurring at a median time of 3 months after transplantation and 18 were solid tumors presenting at a median time of 99 months. Risk factors for solid tumors were chronic GVHD treated with azathioprine and the diagnosis of Fanconi's anemia; azathioprine and irradiation were found to be significant risk factors for those with acquired aplastic anemia. The highest risk of developing a solid tumor was associated with Fanconi's anemia.

*New Solid Cancers after Immunosuppressive Therapy*

Data on solid tumors after immunosuppressive therapy are scarce. In the EBMT study, 8 solid tumors developed in the 860 patients who received immunosuppressive treatment [8]; as compared to the general European population, the risk was 5.15 ($p < 0.001$). Despite the similar incidences of solid tumor after immunosuppression and bone marrow transplantation, transplanted patients have a greater overall risk of developing a malignant solid tumor compared with the general population, due to their younger age. Unpublished results of the German trial comparing ALG, prednisone and cyclosporin showed that in the long term 3 patients developed solid tumors, one of which was certainly a concurrent cancer since it occurred only 3 months after treatment.

## Long-Term Follow-Up after Allogeneic Marrow Transplantation

To provide a long-term perspective of treatment results, the outcome in patients with aplastic anemia transplanted in Seattle and surviving for 2 years after transplantation was recently evaluated by Deeg et al. [14]. With follow-ups of up to 26 years, these patients have an excellent life expectancy and most are doing well. Chronic GVHD, which had developed in 41% of patients, was the most frequent late event and had an impact on survival: 89% of patients without chronic GVHD were expected to survive at 20 years, compared with 69% for those with chronic GVHD. Thirteen of 17 patients who died at 2.5–20.4 years had chronic GVHD; none of the 4 late deaths in patients without chronic GVHD was directly related to transplantation. Risk factors for chronic GVHD were those recognized in earlier studies, i.e. acute GVHD, infusion of viable donor buffy coat cells, and older patient age. Improved supportive care in recent years appears to have increased survival by reducing mortality in the first 2 years after transplantation. Interestingly, patients transplanted before 1978 who developed chronic GVHD and survived for 2 years were as likely to survive as patients without chronic GVHD, presumably because those with the most severe problems died early, i.e. before 2 years.

Chronic GVHD emerged as a risk factor for nearly all long-term complications. Aside from a direct involvement of target organs by GVHD (skin, lungs), treatment of GVHD, especially with steroids, enhanced the likelihood of delayed complications such as cataracts or musculo-skeletal disease. In fact, cataracts and aseptic necrosis occurred exclusively in patients who had received glucocorticoids. On the other hand, pulmonary problems were most frequent in patients with de novo chronic GVHD. This observation suggests the possibility that late institution of GVHD therapy in patients who never had clinically apparent acute GVHD allowed for the development of pulmonary pathology.

The Seattle group has shown previously that patients with aplastic anemia conditioned for transplantation with a nonirradiation regimen were likely to preserve their ability to become pregnant or father normal children. This finding was confirmed in this study, although it is unknown how many of the patients attempted to have children. It is also not clear why transplantation in more recent years was associated with a higher likelihood of posttransplantation pregnancy.

Finally, Deeg et al. [14] also attempted to evaluate the patients' current status by means of self-assessment questionnaires. Neither time from transplantation nor the presence of chronic GVHD had a significant impact on the patients' self-assessment score, although there was a trend for patients with chronic GVHD and for older patients to score lower than patients without GVHD and younger patients. Regardless of GVHD, however, patients generally assessed their quality of life as excellent. By 2 years after transplantation, 83% of the patients were employed or had returned to school; this proportion had increased to 86–90% by 15–20 years.

The present analysis confirms that marrow transplantation offers effective therapy for patients with aplastic anemia. Most patients who survived for at least 2 years after transplantation returned to a productive life. The likelihood was higher in patients without chronic GVHD. The probability of being well and returning to a functionally satisfactory lifestyle was somewhat better than reported for patients transplanted for a malignant disorder. At last follow-up, all patients had normal hematopoiesis derived from donor cells, providing proof that small numbers of stem cells allow for long-term effective hematopoiesis. In contrast to patients given immunosuppressive therapy, none of the transplanted patients developed a new hematologic disorder.

## Long-Term Follow-Up after Immunosuppressive Therapy

In contrast to data reporting long-term outcomes after transplantation, those reporting nonmalignant complications and quality of life after immunosuppressive therapy are scarce. A study by the Hammersmith group demonstrated, however, that nongrafted patients are at increased risk of developing avascular necrosis of bone [22]. A study comparing grafted to nongrafted patients with regard to long-term complications and quality of life could thus be of important clinical value.

## References


1 Schrezenmeier H, Hildebrand A, Rojewski M, Häcker H, Heimpel H, Raghavachar A: Paroxysmal nocturnal haemoglobinuria: A replacement of haematopoietic tissue? Acta Haematol 2000;103:41–48.

2 De Planque MM, Kluinnelemans HC, Van Krieken HJ, Kluin PM, Brand A, Beverstock GC, et al: Evolution of acquired severe aplastic anaemia to myelodysplastic and subsequent leukemia in adults. Br J Haematol 1989;70:55–61.

3 Tichelli A, Gratwohl A, Wursch A, Nissen C, Speck B: Late haematological complications in severe aplastic anaemia. Br J Haematol 1988; 69:413–418.

4 Tichelli A, Gratwohl A, Nissen C, Speck B: Late clonal complications in severe aplastic anemia. Leuk Lymphoma 1994;12:167–175.

5 De Planque MM, Bacigalupo A, Wursch A, Hows J, Devergie A, Frickhofen N, et al: Long-term follow-up of severe aplastic anaemia patients treated with antilymphocyte globulin. Br J Haematol 1989;73:121–126.

6 Paquette RL, Tebyani N, Frane M, Ireland P, Ho WG, Champlin RE, et al: Long-term outcome of aplastic anemia in adults treated with antithymocyte globulin: Comparison with bone marrow transplantation. Blood 1995;85: 283–290.

7 Doney K, Leisenring W, Storb R, Appelbaum FR: Primary treatment of acquired aplastic anemia: Outcomes with bone marrow transplantation and immunosuppressive therapy. Ann Intern Med 1997;126:107–115.

8 Socie G, Henryamar M, Bacigalupo A, Hows J, Tichelli A, Ljungman P, et al: Malignant tumors occurring after treatment of aplastic anemia. N Engl J Med 1993;329:1152–1157.

9 Ohara A, Kojima S, Hamajima N, Tsuchida M, Imashuku S, Ohta S, et al: Myelodysplastic syndrome and acute myelogenous leukemia as a late clonal complication in children with acquired aplastic anemia. Blood 1997;90:1009–1013.

10 Kaito K, Kobayashi M, Katayama T, Masuoka H, Shimada T, Nishiwaki K, et al: Long-term administration of G-CSG for aplastic anaemia is closely related to the early evolution of monosomy 7 MDS in adults. Br J Haematol 1998; 103:297–303.

11 Bacigalupo A, Broccia G, Corda G, Arcese W, Carotenuto M, Gallamini A, et al: Antilymphocyte globulin, cyclosporin, and granulocyte colony-stimulating factor in patients with acquired severe aplastic anemia (SAA): A pilot study of the EBMT SAA Working Party. Blood 1995;85:1348–1353.

12 Rosenfeld SJ, Kimball J, Vining D, Young NS: Intensive immunosuppression with antithymocyte globulin and cyclosporine as treatment for severe acquired aplastic anemia. Blood 1995; 85:3058–3065.

13 Frickhofen N, Schrezenmeier H, Bacigalupo A: Results of European trials of immunosuppression for treatment of aplastic anemia; in Gluckman E, Coulombel L (eds): Ontogeny of Hematopiesis, Aplastic Anemia. Libbey Eurotext 1995, pt 5: Treatment of aplastic anemia, pp 335–345.

14 Deeg HJ, Leisenring W, Storb R, Nims J, Flowers MED, Witherspoon RP, et al: Long-term outcome after marrow transplantation for severe aplastic anemia. Blood 1998;91:3637–3645.

15 Browne PV, Lawler M, Humphries P, McCann SR: Donor-cell leukemia after bone marrow transplantation for severe aplastic anemia. N Engl J Med 1991;325:710–713.

16 Appelbaum F, Barrall J, Storb R, Ramberg R, Doney K, Sale G, et al: Clonal cytogenetic abnormalities in patients with otherwise typical aplastic anemia. Exp Hematol 1987;15: 1134–1139.

17 Mikhailova N, Sessarego M, Fugazza G, Caimo A, Defilippi S, Vanlint MT, et al: Cytogenetic abnormalities in patients with severe aplastic anemia. Haematologica 1996;81:418–422.

18 Yamazaki E, Kanamori H, Taguchi J, Harano H, Mohri H, Okubo T: The evidence of clonal evolution with monosomy 7 in aplastic anemia following granulocyte colony-stimulating factor using the polymerase chain reaction. Blood Cells Mol Dis 1997;23:213–218.

19 Socié G, Henryamar M, Cosset JM, Devergie A, Girinski T, Gluckman E: Increased incidence of solid malignant tumors after bone marrow transplantation for severe aplastic anemia. Blood 1991;78:277–279.

20 Witherspoon RP, Storb R, Pepe M, Longton G, Sullivan KM: Cumulative incidence of secondary solid malignant tumors in aplastic anemia given marrow grafts after conditioning with chemotherapy alone. Blood 1991;79:289–291.

21 Deeg HJ, Socié G, Schoch G, Henryamar M, Witherspoon RP, Devergie A, et al: Malignancies after marrow transplantation for aplastic anemia and Fanconi anemia: A joint Seattle and Paris analysis of results in 700 patients. Blood 1996;87:386–392.

22 Marsh JCW, Zomas A, Hows JM, Chapple M, Gordonsmith EC: Avascular necrosis after treatment of aplastic anaemia with antilymphocyte globulin and high-dose methylprednisolone. Br J Haematol 1993;84:731–735.

Acta Hæmatologica

Acta Haematol 2000;103:55–62

# Predictive Factors for Cure after Immunosuppressive Therapy of Aplastic Anemia

Romaine Viollier André Tichelli

Hematological Laboratory, Department of Central Laboratory and Division of Hematology, Department of Internal Medicine, University Hospitals, Basel, Switzerland

**Key Words**
Antilymphocyte globulin · Aplastic anemia · Immunosuppression · Relapse

**Abstract**
In a previous study, we evaluated efficacy of repeated antilymphocyte globulin (ALG) treatment for patients with severe aplastic anemia not responding to an initial ALG treatment or relapsing after initial response to ALG. We now searched in the same cohort of patients for differences between patients who responded to treatment and remained free of complications and those who relapsed or developed a clonal complication. From 107 patients surviving for more than 1 year after immunosuppression, 34 remained free from complications after the first course of ALG, and 73 presented an event defined as relapse of aplastic anemia, development of a clonal complication such as paroxysmal nocturnal hemoglobinuria, myelodysplastic syndrome or leukemia, or appearance of a solid tumor. We compared these two groups for survival, clinical performance and blood counts during follow-up. Survival probability was 93% for the event-free patients, and 55% for the patients with a complication event ($p = 0.0003$). Event-free patients had a higher incidence of complete remission (71%), were more often free of immunosuppressive treatment (79%) and independent of transfusions (100%), and had a higher Karnofsky score (91% with a score ≥90%) as compared to the group with events (29, 37, 67, 48%; $p \leq 0.0002$). At 1 and 3 years, event-free patients had significantly higher leukocyte and neutrophil counts, as compared to patients with a complication ($p < 0.05$). However, at 3 and 5 years, event-free patients had borderline higher platelet counts ($p = 0.056$, $p = 0.078$) and hemoglobin ($p = 0.097$, $p = 0.061$). The coefficient of variation as an expression of the variability of the results in each group was systematically lower at 3, 5 and 10 years in the group of event-free patients. Despite some differences between the two groups, our data support the hypothesis that patients with long-lasting remissions should not be considered as definitively cured of aplastic anemia.



## Introduction

Stem cell transplantation or treatment with antilymphocyte globulin (ALG) therapy are the treatments of choice for patients with aplastic anemia. Both modalities have improved the outcome [1–6]. Sixty to eighty percent

KARGER
Fax + 41 61 306 12 34
E-Mail karger@karger.ch
www.karger.com


0001–5792/00/1031–0055$17.50/0

Accessible online at:
www.karger.com/journals/aha

André Tichelli, MD
Hematological Laboratory
Department of Central Laboratory University Hospitals
Petersgraben 4, CH–4031 Basel (Switzerland)
Tel. +41 61 265 42 56, Fax +41 61 265 44 50, E-Mail Atichelli@uhbs.ch

**Table 1.** Characteristics of the 107 patients with aplastic anemia treated with ALG, and comparison between the group of patients presenting an event during their follow-up with those not presenting an event

| | All patients | Patients with no event | Patients with an event | p value |
|---|---|---|---|---|
| Number | 107 | 34 | 73 | |
| Age, years | | | | |
| Median (range) | 22 (1–71) | 22 (1–62) | 22 (2–71) | n.s. |
| Gender | | | | |
| Males | 59 (55%) | 16 (47%) | 43 (59%) | n.s. |
| Etiology | | | | |
| Idiopathic | 87 (81%) | 25 (74%) | 62 (85%) | |
| Viral | 6 (6%) | 3 (9%) | 3 (4%) | n.s. |
| Drug | 13 (12%) | 6 (17%) | 7 (10%) | |
| Others | 1 (1%) | 0 | 1 (1%) | |
| Severity | | | | |
| Moderate | 35 (33%) | 8 (24%) | 27 (37%) | |
| Severe | 47 (44%) | 14 (41%) | 33 (45%) | 0.048[1] |
| Very severe | 25 (23%) | 12 (35%) | 13 (18%) | |
| Follow-up, months | | | | |
| Median (range) | 132 (12–263) | 142 (1–254) | 129 (1–263) | n.s. |
| Blood counts before therapy | | | | |
| Leukocytes, $\times 10^9$/l | 2.2 (0–6.00) | 1.8 (0.1–5.4) | 2.5 (0–6.00) | 0.01 |
| Neutrophils, $\times 10^9$/l | 0.42 (0–2.1) | 0.31 (0–1.47) | 0.43 (0–2.1) | n.s. |
| Platelets, $\times 10^9$/l | 10 (1–75) | 10 (1–75) | 9 (1–43) | n.s. |
| Reticulocytes, $\times 10^9$/l | 10 (186) | 5 (0–44) | 12 (186) | n.s. |

[1] Comparison between groups of patients with very severe aplastic anemia.

of patients with newly diagnosed acquired aplastic anemia respond to the treatment. However, there are basic differences between the two treatment groups. Hematologic reconstitution is usually fast and complete after stem cell transplantation. In contrast, recovery often takes several months after ALG treatment [7]. Immunosuppression, although allowing autologous reconstitution of hematopoiesis, leaves the patient with a fragile bone marrow prone to the development of a clonal complication. These observations support the fact that patients with aplastic anemia are usually not cured of their disease after treatment with immunosuppression. It is therefore not surprising that relapse of aplastic anemia and late hematological complications, such as paroxysmal nocturnal hemoglobinuria (PNH), myelodysplastic syndromes (MDS) or leukemia may occur [8–14].

Complete remission and survival of leukemia are usually closely related. Curative treatment is defined as the proportion of patients who survive beyond the time after which the risk of treatment failure approaches zero. For aplastic anemia, the situation is much more complex. Survival is no longer the unique criterion of success. Although relapses after an initial response to immunosuppression are common [15, 16], they are a treatable condition and may even respond repeatedly. Hematological recovery and survival at 10 years after repeated treatment with ALG are comparable to results in patients treated only once [13, 16–20]. On the other hand, late clonal complications can interfere with survival of patients with aplastic anemia.

In a previous study, we evaluated the efficacy of repeated ALG treatment in patients with severe aplastic anemia not responding to an initial ALG treatment or relapsing after initial response to ALG [21]. One hundred and thirty-nine consecutive patients with newly diagnosed aplastic anemia were treated with ALG between 1976 and 1995. Eighty-nine patients (64%) responded to a first course of ALG, while 50 patients did not become independent of transfusion. Of the 89 responders, 66 remained relapse free. These data suggested that some of the patients never relapsing might be cured of their disease after immunosuppression. We addressed this hypothesis in the present study. Therefore, we reevaluated the same cohort, and looked for a difference between patients who responded to treatment and remained free of any event and those who relapsed or developed a clonal complication. The ultimate goal of this analysis is to find a predictive factor of cure.

## Patients and Methods

*Patients*

We compared patients who remained in long-term remission with patients presenting any type of complication during their follow-up. For this study, we used the cohort of 139 patients treated between 1976 and 1996, who had been evaluated in the study on repeated treatment with ALG [21]. Of these 137 patients, 107 patients surviving the first year of treatment, and updated as of 1 January 1999 were included (table 1). Patients with aplastic anemia as defined by the criteria of Camitta et al. [22] and Bacigalupo et al. [1] have been treated uniformly since 1976. Patients younger than 40 years of age with an HLA-matched sibling donor were transplanted; older patients and patients without an HLA-identical sibling donor were treated with ALG. The treatment protocol and overall results were published previously [23, 24].

*Definitions and Factors Analyzed*

Patients were classified into two groups: those who remained free of complications after the first course of ALG, and those who presented an event, defined as relapse of the aplastic anemia, development of a clonal complication, such as PNH, MDS or leukemia, or the appearance of a solid tumor. We compared clinical data and peripheral blood counts (leukocytes, neutrophils, platelets, reticulocytes, hemoglobin and mean corpuscular volume, MCV) in both groups of patients at diagnosis, and at 1, 3, 5 and 10 years after initial immunosuppressive treatment, at the time of the best remission state, as well as at the last follow-up observation. The following clinical data were considered: type of response to immunosuppression, need for continuous treatment (cyclosporin A, repeated ALG, androgens, steroids, any specific treatment for PNH, MDS, leukemia or solid tumors), independence from transfusion as well as the Karnofsky score. Complete remission was defined as independence from transfusion and normal blood counts (hemoglobin ≥13 g/dl for males, ≥12 g/dl for females; platelet counts $\geq 150 \times 10^9$/l, granulocyte counts $\geq 1.5 \times 10^9$/l). The definition of partial remission included independence from transfusion as an invariable criterion, but varied according to the initial severity of the disease. For the group with severe disease, partial remission was obtained when the definition of severe aplastic anemia was no longer met. In case of nonsevere aplastic anemia, partial remission was achieved when one cell line showed doubling or normalization. PNH, MDS or leukemia in patients with aplastic anemia were defined in detail previously [14].

*Statistical Analysis*

Group differences were analyzed by the Mann-Whitney U test for continuous variables, and the Pearson $\chi^2$ test for categorical variables. Survival probabilities were estimated by the method of Kaplan and Meier [25]. The log-rank test was used to compare survival [26]. For all statistical analyses, p values $\leq 0.05$ were considered significant. Statistical analysis was performed by using the SPSS statistical program (SPSS for Windows, release 8.0, SPSS, Inc., Chicago, Ill., USA).

## Results

Clinical characteristics of the two groups of patients are shown in table 1. Median age, gender, etiology of the aplastic anemia, and median follow-up time were comparable between the groups. Interestingly, however, the group of patients never presenting any complication included more individuals with very severe aplastic anemia, and lower median leukocyte counts at diagnosis ($p = 0.01$).

*Survival and Probability of an Event*

From the 107 patients, 34 (32%) remained free of an event, 73 (68%) developed an event, as defined above. As of 1 January 1999, 76 (71%) of 107 patients surviving for more than 1 year were alive. Of the 34 event-free patients 33 (97%) were alive, and 1 patient died of cardiac insufficiency, unrelated to aplastic anemia or its treatment. In the group with an event, 43 of 73 patients (59%) were alive and 30 had died (disease related [n = 11]; complication-related [n = 14]; treatment-related [n = 4], and unrelated to disease or treatment [n = 1]). Survival probability for the entire cohort was 66 ± 5% at 15 years (table 2). For the event-free patients, it was 93 ± 6%, for the patients with an event, 55 ± 7% ($p = 0.0003$) (fig. 1). The cumulative probability of developing an event at 20 years after immunosuppressive treatment was 77 ± 5% (fig. 2). Differences in the status of the best remission ever achieved were observed between the groups. The event-free patients had a higher incidence of complete remission (82%), as compared to the patients with an event (55%; $p = 0.01$). There was a delay before the best remission state was obtained in the event-free group. The median time to obtain the best remission was 35 months, as compared to 12 months for patients with an event ($p = 0.002$) (fig. 3).

*Clinical Performance during Follow-Up*

Considering that complete remission should correlate with an optimal clinical performance, we compared the need for continuous treatment, independence from transfusion and the Karnofsky scores of both groups. Clinical performance at the time of last follow-up showed significant differences (table 2). Event-free patients had a higher incidence of complete remission (71%), were more often free of immunosuppressive treatment (79%) and independent of transfusions (100%), and had higher Karnofsky scores (91% patients with a score ≥90%), as compared to the group with events (29, 37, 67, 48%; $p \leq 0.0002$).

**Table 2.** Clinical performance of the 107 patients with aplastic anemia at the time of the best remission state and during last follow-up: comparison between the group of patients presenting an event during their follow-up with those not presenting an event

| | All patients | Patients with no event | Patients with an event | p value |
|---|---|---|---|---|
| Number | 107 | 34 | 73 | |
| Alive | 76 (71%) | 33 (97%) | 43 (59%) | <0.001 |
| Probability of being alive at 15 years | 66±5% | 93±6% | 55±7% | 0.0003 |
| Splenectomy | 65 (61%) | 17 (50%) | 48 (66%) | 0.12 |
| Best remission state | | | | |
| Complete remission | 68 (63%) | 28 (82%) | 40 (55%) | 0.01 |
| Partial remission | 34 (32%) | 6 (18%) | 28 (38%) | |
| No response | 5 (5%) | 0 | 5 (7%) | |
| Time to best remission state, months | | | | |
| Median (range) | 13 (3–185) | 35 (3–171) | 12 (3–185) | 0.002 |
| Remission state at last follow-up | | | | |
| Complete remission | 45 (42%) | 24 (71%) | 21 (29%) | |
| Partial remission | 25 (24%) | 10 (29%) | 15 (20%) | <0.001 |
| No response | 10 (9%) | 0 | 10 (14%) | |
| Events | 27 (25%) | 0 | 27 (37%) | |
| Patients without immunosuppressive treatment at last follow-up | 52 (50%) | 26 (79%) | 26 (37%) | <0.001 |
| Independence from transfusion at last follow-up | 83 (78%) | 34 (100%) | 49 (67%) | <0.0001 |
| Patients with Karnofsky ≥90% | 66 (62%) | 31 (91%) | 35 (48%) | <0.001 |
| Karnofsky score, % | | | | |
| Median (range) | 90 (30–100) | 100 (50–100) | 80 (30–100) | <0.001 |

At the predetermined observation times, the difference between the groups was not obvious. One and 3 years after immunosuppression, no significant differences were observed (table 3). At most, the event-free patients had a slightly higher remission rate, as compared to patients with an event ($p = 0.089$, $p = 0.063$). The situation was more explicit at 5 and 10 years after treatment: All event-free patients were in remission and independent of transfusion ($p > 0.05$), and 91 and 80% of the patients had a Karnofsky score of 90 or 100%. At 10 years, 83% of this group of patients were free of treatment, as compared to 42% in the group with an event ($p = 0.012$).

*Blood Counts during Follow-Up*

Blood counts at 1, 3, 5, and 10 years after immunosuppression were compared between the groups (table 4). At 1 and 3 years, event-free patients had significantly higher leukocyte and neutrophil counts as compared to patients with an event ($p < 0.05$). At 3 and 5 years, event-free patients had borderline higher platelet counts ($p = 0.056$, $p = 0.078$) and hemoglobin ($p = 0.097$, $p = 0.061$). There was no difference for the other parameters at the respective observation times. At 10 years after immunosuppression, none of the blood counts showed a statistical difference between the groups.

To express the variability of the results in each group statistically, we used the coefficient of variation, which compares the spread of the results. However, the coefficient of variation is not only determined by the statistical variation, but it is also dependent on the counting number. With increasing numbers, the coefficient of variation decreases. For blood counts after the first year, no clear pattern was observed between the groups (table 4). However, at 3, 5 and 10 years, and despite the lower counts in the event-free group, these patients systematically showed lower coefficients of variation.

## Discussion

This study demonstrates that about one third of the patients surviving the first year after immunosuppression will have a long-term event-free survival, i.e. a survival without relapse of the aplastic anemia, or the development of a secondary disease, such as PNH, MDS, leuke-

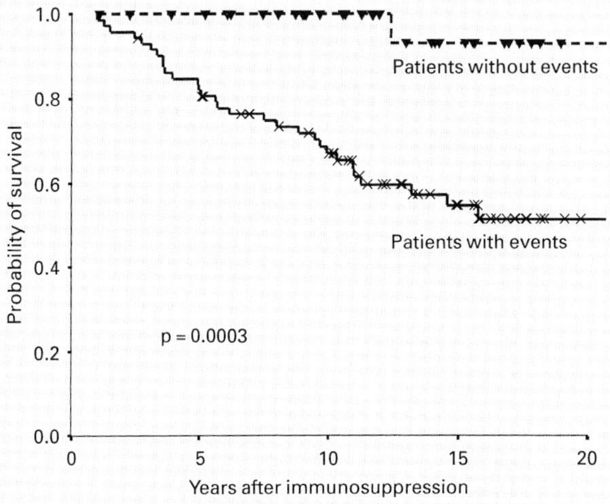


1

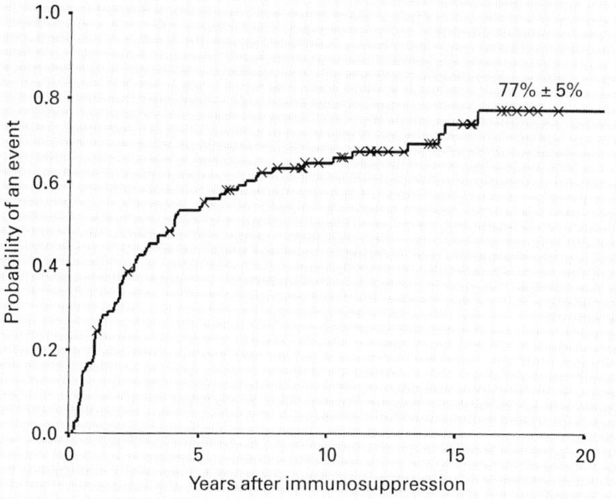


2

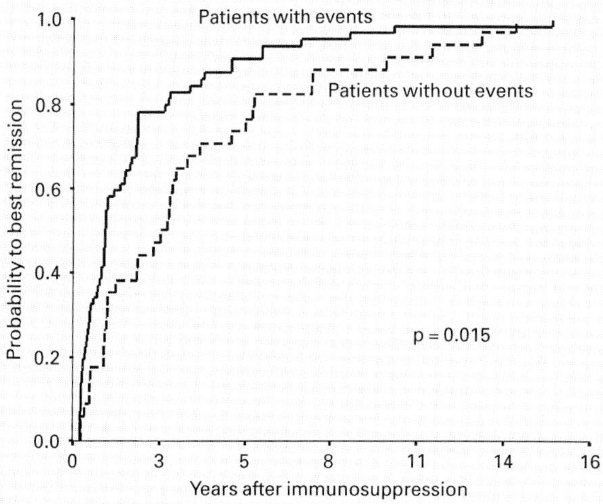


3

**Fig. 1.** Probability of survival according to Kaplan and Meier of the 107 patients with aplastic anemia, surviving the first year of immunosuppressive treatment. Comparison between event-free patients (– – –) and patients presenting an event (——).

**Fig. 2.** Cumulative probability of developing an event after immunosuppressive treatment of the 107 patients with aplastic anemia, surviving the first year of immunosuppressive treatment. The event was defined as a complication occurring during the follow-up, such as a relapse of aplastic anemia, or the development of PNH, MDS, leukemia, or solid tumors.

**Fig. 3.** Cumulative probability of obtaining the best remission state after immunosuppressive treatment of the 107 patients with aplastic anemia, surviving the first year of immunosuppressive treatment. Comparison between event-free patients (– – –) and patients presenting an event (——).

mia, or solid tumor. The survival of this particular group of aplastic anemia patients exceeds 90% at 15 years, as compared to 55% for patients presenting an event. Is it now possible to extrapolate, that (1) event-free patients can be considered as cured after immunosuppressive treatment, and that (2) it should be possible to identify the good risk patients early, where eventually a stem cell transplantation would be unnecessary?

The present results show that patients of the event-free group more often normalize their peripheral blood counts, become independent of transfusions, and present a higher clinical performance rate. Interestingly, the delay to obtain the best remission state is significantly longer, as compared to the patients developing an event subsequently. Two reasons could explain this delay in event-free patients. As previously reported, a rapid recovery is associated with a higher risk of relapsing aplastic anemia [27]. Additionally, we also observed that patients eventually achieving complete remission, often remained in partial remission over months or even years.

There is no difference in clinical performance during the first and third year after immunosuppressive treatment between groups of patients with and without an event. At 5 years event-free patients clearly improved; all of them were in complete remission and independent of transfusions, and 91% of them had a Karnofsky score of 90 or 100%. However, two thirds of the event-free patients at 5 years, and 17% at 10 years still were on cyclosporin A or androgens, which was not different from the group with complications. This probably rather reflects

**Table 3.** Clinical performance of the 107 patients with aplastic anemia at 1, 3, 5 and 10 years after treatment with ALG: comparison between the group of patients presenting an event during their follow-up with those not presenting an event

| | All patients | Patients with no event | Patients with an event | p value |
|---|---|---|---|---|
| *At 1 year* | 91 | 27 | 64 | |
| Remission state | | | | |
| Remission | 76 (83%) | 25 (93%) | 51 (80%) | |
| No response | 9 (10%) | 2 (7%) | 7 (11%) | 0.089 |
| Event | 6 (7%) | 0 | 6 (9%) | |
| Free of treatment | 3/90 (3%) | 1/26 (4%) | 2/64 (3%) | n.s. |
| Transfusion independence | 78 (85%) | 25 (89%) | 53 (83%) | n.s. |
| Karnofsky score ≥ 90% | 71 (78%) | 23 (85%) | 48 (75%) | n.s. |
| *At 3 years* | 93 | 26 | 67 | |
| Remission state | | | | |
| Remission | 82 (88%) | 25 (96%) | 57 (85%) | |
| No response | 3 (3%) | 1 (4%) | 2 (3%) | 0.063 |
| Event | 8 (9%) | 0 | 8 (12%) | |
| Free of treatment | 89/98 (91%) | 28/31 (91%) | 61/67 (91%) | n.s. |
| Transfusion independence | 82 (89%) | 25 (96%) | 57 (86%) | n.s. |
| Karnofsky score ≥ 90% | 77 (84%) | 24 (92%) | 53 (80%) | n.s. |
| *At 5 years* | 80 | 23 | 57 | |
| Remission state | | | | |
| Remission | 68 (85%) | 23 (100%) | 45 (79%) | |
| No response | 1 (1%) | 0 | 1 (2%) | 0.011 |
| Event | 11 (14%) | 0 | 11 (19%) | |
| Free of treatment | 21/72 (29%) | 6/15 (33%) | 15/54 (28%) | n.s. |
| Transfusion independence | 73 (91%) | 23 (100%) | 50 (88%) | 0.025 |
| Karnofsky score ≥ 90% | 64 (80%) | 21 (91%) | 43 (75%) | 0.087 |
| *At 10 years* | 55 | 15 | 40 | |
| Remission state | | | | |
| Remission | 44 (80%) | 15 (100%) | 29 (72%) | |
| No response | 1 (2%) | 0 | 1 (3%) | 0.018 |
| Event | 10 (18%) | 0 | 10 (25%) | |
| Free of treatment | 25/48 (54%) | 10/15 (83%) | 15/36 (42%) | 0.012 |
| Transfusion independence | 48 (87%) | 15 (100%) | 33 (82%) | 0.028 |
| Karnofsky score ≥ 90% | 39 (71%) | 12 (80%) | 27 (67%) | n.s. |

the tendency in clinical habits of many treating centers, which are reluctant to withdraw immunosuppression even in patients with complete remission, because of the fear of a relapse.

Peripheral blood counts during follow-up showed statistical differences between the groups, despite the consistent overlap. Overall, event-free patients presented higher leukocyte and neutrophil counts at the first and third year, and higher platelet counts and hemoglobin at the third and fifth year after immunosuppressive treatment. Five and 10 years after treatment, the spread of the results in the event-free group of patients, expressed as a coefficient of variation, was lower. This can be interpreted as an indirect sign for a higher number of patients with a normalized blood count.

Overall, these data show that many patients with aplastic anemia can have blood values allowing a nearly normal life, independent of their initial response and the development of a complication. Despite differences between event-free patients and patients presenting a complication during their follow-up, there is no clear cut-off between the groups. Not all event-free patients normalize their blood counts even at 10 years, and some of them clearly retain stigmata of the disease, such as persisting macrocytosis, morphological abnormalities of the bone marrow, or a decreased in vitro proliferation capacity as

**Table 4.** Blood counts of the 107 patients with aplastic anemia at 1, 3, 5 and 10 years after immunosuppression: comparison between the group of patients presenting an event during their follow-up with those not presenting an event

| | All patients | Patients with no event | Patients with an event | p value | CV (%)* no | CV (%)* yes |
|---|---|---|---|---|---|---|
| *Blood counts at 1 year* | | | | | | |
| Number | 90 | 26 | 64 | | | |
| Leukocytes, $\times 10^9$/l | 4.2 (1.4–13.6) | 4.6 (2.3–13.6) | 3.9 (1.4–8.1) | 0.036 | 47 | 36 |
| Neutrophils, $\times 10^9$/l | 1.7 (0.13–8.1) | 2.1 (0.9–8.1) | 1.6 (0.13–4.5) | 0.03 | 67 | 59 |
| Platelets, $\times 10^9$/l | 88 (9–512) | 107 (18–386) | 85 (9–512) | n.s. | 71 | 91 |
| Hemoglobin, g/dl | 13.5 (8–17) | 13.6 (5.7–16) | 13.3 (5.7–17) | n.s. | 16 | 23 |
| Reticulocytes, $\times 10^9$/l | 52 (2–212) | 53 (2–212) | 53 (2–212) | n.s. | 66 | 58 |
| MCV, fl | 103 (81–128) | 106 (85–123) | 103 (81–128) | n.s. | 9 | 10 |
| *Blood counts at 3 years* | | | | | | |
| Number | 92 | 26 | 66 | | | |
| Leukocytes, $\times 10^9$/l | 4.9 (1.3–12.4) | 5.8 (2.0–10.4) | 4.5 (1.3–12.4) | 0.03 | 38 | 48 |
| Neutrophils, $\times 10^9$/l | 2.1 (0.08–7.6) | 2.3 (0.88–5.9) | 1.9 (0.08–7.6) | 0.015 | 47 | 71 |
| Platelets, $\times 10^9$/l | 139 (6–506) | 165 (46–399) | 118 (6–506) | 0.056 | 48 | 70 |
| Hemoglobin, g/dl | 13.7 (4.9–18) | 13.9 (8–16) | 13.3 (4.9–18) | 0.097 | 14 | 24 |
| Reticulocytes, $\times 10^9$/l | 56 (2–176) | 43 (6–150) | 59 (2–176) | n.s. | 71 | 62 |
| MCV, fl | 101 (85–126) | 102 (85–125) | 101 (85–126) | n.s. | 10 | 8 |
| *Blood counts at 5 years* | | | | | | |
| Number | 80 | 23 | 57 | | | |
| Leukocytes, $\times 10^9$/l | 5.0 (0.3–20.6) | 5.4 (2.6–11.5) | 4.9 (0.3–20.6) | n.s. | 38 | 59 |
| Neutrophils, $\times 10^9$/l | 2.1 (0.13–19) | 2.6 (1.0–5.9) | 2.0 (0.13–19) | n.s. | 53 | 142 |
| Platelets, $\times 10^9$/l | 149 (2–396) | 170 (53–396) | 127 (2–351) | 0.078 | 46 | 72 |
| Hemoglobin, g/dl | 13.4 (5–17) | 13.6 (11–16) | 13.4 (5–17) | 0.061 | 11 | 22 |
| Reticulocytes, $\times 10^9$/l | 52 (2–588) | 53 (2–90) | 48 (4–588) | n.s. | 50 | 180 |
| MCV, fl | 101 (85–131) | 99 (88–117) | 102 (85–131) | n.s. | 8 | 11 |
| *Blood counts at 10 years* | | | | | | |
| Number | 53 | 15 | 38 | | | |
| Leukocytes, $\times 10^9$/l | 4.9 (1.3–11.4) | 4.9 (3.9–10.4) | 4.9 (1.3–11.4) | n.s. | 35 | 43 |
| Neutrophils, $\times 10^9$/l | 2.5 (0.33–7.6) | 2.6 (1.5–4.9) | 2.4 (0.33–7.6) | 0.076 | 36 | 64 |
| Platelets, $\times 10^9$/l | 163 (10–408) | 166 (94–408) | 164 (10–362) | n.s. | 44 | 65 |
| Hemoglobin, g/dl | 13.6 (5.7–17) | 14.4 (8–16) | 13.4 (5.7–17) | n.s. | 14 | 24 |
| Reticulocytes, $\times 10^9$/l | 56 (9–250) | 57 (9–95) | 55 (30–250) | n.s. | 41 | 63 |
| MCV, fl | 100 (82–123) | 99 (8714) | 100 (82–123) | n.s. | 7 | 10 |

CV = Coefficient of variation; no = patients without an event; yes = patients with an event.

well as a low capacity to initiate long-term bone marrow cultures [7, 28–31]. On the other hand, patients can obtain a long-term remission even after a relapse of the aplastic anemia [21]. The hope, that the first event of a patient presenting a complication would occur within few years after immunosuppressive treatment, and thereby allow early identification of the patients at risk could not be sustained. Indeed, the probability of developing a first event at 15 years increases up to 77%, without showing signs of reaching a plateau.

In conclusion, despite some differences between the two groups, our data support the hypothesis that patients with long-lasting remission should not be considered as definitively cured of aplastic anemia. So far, there is no marker allowing to identify patients who will not develop a late complication after immunosuppression. Therefore, younger patients with an HLA-matched sibling donor should continue to be considered for stem cell transplantation as first-line treatment.


## Acknowledgment

We thank Alexandra Wodnar-Filipowicz and Alois Gratwohl for a critical review of the manuscript.

## References


1 Bacigalupo A, Hows J, Gluckman E, Nissen C, Marsh JCW, Van Lint MT, Congiu M, De Planque MM, Ernst P, McCann S, Ragavashar A, Frickhofen N, Würsch A, Marmont AM, Gordon-Smith EC: Bone marrow transplantation (BMT) versus immunosuppression for the treatment of severe aplastic anaemia: A report of the EBMT SAA Working Party. Br J Haematol 1988;70:177–182.

2 Doney K, Leisenring W, Storb R, Appelbaum FR: Primary treatment of acquired aplastic anemia: Outcomes with bone marrow transplantation and immunosuppressive therapy. Ann Intern Med 1997;126:107–115.

3 Frickhofen N, Kaltwasser JP, Schrezenmeier H, Ragavashar A, Vogt HG, Herrmann F, Freund M, Meusers P, Salama A, Heimpel H: Treatment of aplastic anemia with antilymphocyte globulin and methylprednisolone with or without cyclosporine. N Engl J Med 1991;324:1297–1304.

4 Paquette RL, Tebyani N, Frane M, Ireland P, Ho WG, Champlin RE, Nimer SD: Long-term outcome of aplastic anemia in adults treated with antithymocyte globulin: Comparison with bone marrow transplantation. Blood 1995;85:283–290.

5 Passweg JR, Socié G, Hinterberger W, Bacigalupo A, Biggs JC, Camitta BM, Champlin RE, Gale RP, Gluckman E, Gordon-Smith EC, Hows JM, Klein JP, Nugent ML, Pasquini R, Rowlings PA, Speck B, Tichelli A, Zhang MJ, Horowitz MM, Bortin MM: Bone marrow transplantation for severe aplastic anemia: Has outcome improved? Blood 1997;90:858–864.

6 Storb R, Leisenring W, Anasetti C, Appelbaum FR, Buckner CD, Bensinger WI, Chauncey T, Clift RA, Deeg HJ, Doney KC, Flowers MED, Hansen JA, Martin PJ, Sanders KM, Witherspoon RP: Long-term follow-up of allogeneic marrow transplants in patients with aplastic anemia conditioned by cyclophosphamide combined with antithymocyte globulin. Blood 1997;89:3890–3891.

7 Nissen C, Gratwohl A, Tichelli A, Stebler C, Wursch A, Moser Y, dalle Carbonare V, Signer E, Buser M, Ritz R: Gender and response to antilymphocyte globulin (ALG) for severe aplastic anaemia. Br J Haematol 1993;83:319–325.

8 De Planque MM, Kluin-Nelemans HC, Van Krieken HJM, Kluin PM, Brand A, Beverstock GC, Willemze R, Van Rood JJ: Evolution of acquired severe aplastic anaemia to myelodysplastic and subsequent leukaemia in adults. Br J Haematol 1988;70:55.

9 De Planque MM, Kluin-Nelemans HC, van Krieken HJ, Kluin PM, Brand A, Beverstock GC, Willemze R, van Rood JJ: Evolution of acquired severe aplastic anaemia to myelodysplasia and subsequent leukaemia in adults. Br J Haematol 1988;70:55–62.

10 Marsh JC, Geary CG: Is aplastic anaemia a pre-leukaemic disorder? (editorial). Br J Haematol 1991;77:447–452.

11 Najean Y, Haguenauer O: Long-term (5 to 20 years) evolution of nongrafted aplastic anemias. The Cooperative Group for the Study of Aplastic and Refractory Anemias. Blood 1990;76:2222–2228.

12 Narayanan MN, Geary CG, Freemont AJ, Kendra JR: Long-term follow-up of aplastic anaemia. Br J Haematol 1994;86:837–843.

13 Socié G, Henry-Amar M, Bacigalupo A, Hows J, Tichelli A, Ljungman P, McCann SR, Frickhofen N, Van't Veer-Korthof E, Gluckman E: Malignant tumors occurring after treatment of aplastic anemia. European Bone Marrow Transplantation-Severe Aplastic Anaemia Working Party. N Engl J Med 1993;329:1152–1157.

14 Tichelli A, Gratwohl A, Würsch A, Nissen C, Speck B: Late haematological complications in severe aplastic anaemia. Br J Haematol 1988;69:413–418.

15 Marsh JC, Gordon-Smith EC: Treatment of aplastic anaemia with antilymphocyte globulin and cyclosporin. Int J Hematol 1995;62:133–144.

16 Rosenfeld SJ, Kimball J, Vining D, Young NS: Intensive immunosuppression with antithymocyte globulin and cyclosporine as treatment for severe acquired aplastic anemia. Blood 1995;85:3058–3065.

17 Schrezenmeier H, Hinterberger-Fischer M, Hows J, Ljungman P, Locascuilli A, Marin P, Marsh JC, McCann S, den Ottolander GJ, Ragavashar A, Socie G, Tichelli A, Van't Veer-Korthof E, Bacigalupo A, for the EMBT SAA Working Party. Second immunosuppressive treatment of patients with aplastic anemia not responding to the first course of immunosuppression: A report from the Working Party on Severe Aplastic Anemia of the EBMT (abstract). Bone Marrow Transplant 1998;15(suppl 2):S10–S10.

18 Means RT Jr, Krantz SB, Dessypris EN, Lukens JN, Niblack GD, Greer JP, Flexner JM, Stein RS: Re-treatment of aplastic anemia with antithymocyte globulin or antilymphocyte serum. Am J Med 1988;84:678–682.

19 Marsh JC, Socie G, Schrezenmeier H, Tichelli A, Gluckman E, Ljungman P, McCann SR, Raghavachar A, Marin P, Hows JM: Haemopoietic growth factors in aplastic anaemia: A cautionary note. European Bone Marrow Transplant Working Party for Severe Aplastic Anaemia (see comments). Lancet 1994;344:172–173.

20 Marsh JCW, Gordon-Smith EC: The role of antilymphocyte globulin in the treatment of chronic acquired bone marrow failure. Blood Rev 1988;2:141–148.

21 Tichelli A, Passweg JR, Nissen C, Bargetzi M, Hoffmann T, Wodnar-Filipowicz A, Signer E, Speck B, Gratwohl A: Repeated treatment with horse antilymphocyte globulin for severe aplastic anaemia. Br J Haematol 1998;100:393–400.

22 Camitta BM, Thomas ED, Nathan DG, Santos G, Gordon-Smith EC, Gale RP, Rappeport JM, Storb R: Severe aplastic anemia: A prospective study of the effect of early marrow transplantation on acute mortality. Blood 1976;48:63–70.

23 Speck B, Gratwohl A, Nissen C, Leibundgut U, Ruggero O, Osterwalder B, Burri HP, Cornu P, Jeannet M: Treatment of severe aplastic anaemia with antilymphocyte globuline or bone marrow transplantation. Br Med J 1981;282:860–863.

24 Speck B, Gratwohl A, Nissen C, Osterwalder B, Würsch A, Tichelli A, Lori A, Reusser P, Jeannet M, Signer E: Treatment of severe aplastic anemia. Exp Hematol 1986;14:126–132.

25 Kaplan EL, Meier P: Nonparametric estimation from incomplete observations. J Am Stat Assoc 1958;53:457–481.

26 Peto R, Pike MC, Armitage P, Breslow NE, Cox DR, Howard SV, Mantel N, McPherson K, Peto J, Smith PG: Design and analysis of randomized clinical trials requiring prolonged observation of each patient. Br J Cancer 1977;35:1–39.

27 Schrezenmeier H, Marin P, Raghavachar A, McCann S, Hows J, Gluckman E, Nissen C, van't Veer-Korthof ET, Ljungman P, Hinterberger W, Van Lint MT, Frickhofen N, Bacigalupo A, for the EBMT SAA Working Party: Relapse of aplastic anaemia after immunosuppressive treatment: A report from the European Bone Marrow Transplantation Group SAA Working Party. Br J Haematol 1993;85:371–377.

28 De Planque MM, Brand A, Kluin-Nelemans HC, Eernisse JG, van der Burgh F, Natarajan AT, Beverstock GC, Zwaan FE, Willemze R, van Rood JJ: Haematopoietic and immunologic abnormalities in severe aplastic anaemia patients treated with antithymocyte globulin. Br J Haematol 1989;71:421–430.

29 Marsh JCW, Hows J, Bryett KA, Al-Hashimi S, Fairhead SM, Gordon-Smith EC: Survival after antithymocyte globulin therapy for aplastic anemia depends on disease severity. Blood 1987;70:1046–1052.

30 Tichelli A, Gratwohl A, Nissen C, Signer E, Stebler Gysi Ch, Speck B: Morphology in patients with severe aplastic anemia treated with antilymphocyte globulin. Blood 1992;80:337–345.

31 Marsh JC, Chang J, Testa NG, Hows J, Dexter TM: The hematopoietic defect in aplastic anemia assessed by long-term marrow culture. Blood 1990;76:1–10.

Acta Hæmatologica

Acta Haematol 2000;103:63–64

A Case Report:

# Living with Severe Aplastic Anaemia for 22 Years

## A Patient Tells His Story (Supplemented with Information from the Haematology Clinic Basel, Switzerland)

Ernst Kienle  Catherine Nissen

Haematology Clinic Basel, Basel, Switzerland

Ernst Kienle: In 1977, feeling progessively tired, I was diagnosed with aplastic anaemia at the age of 22 years. My local doctor referred me to Prof. Speck in Basel, Switzerland, who took care of me until his death, in 1998.

I was given bone marrow *(Comment: E.K. was treated with a first course of antilymphocyte globulin, followed by an infusion of HLA-haplotype-matched bone marrow from his brother. At that time, and for the following years, antilymphocyte globulin was used to induce micro-engraftment of mismatched bone marrow).*

My blood values gradually normalised *(which, at the time, suggested that it was the combination of antilymphocyte globulin and mismatched marrow that induced autologous haematopoietic recovery).*

In 1984, as my blood values deteriorated, I was given a second course of antilymphocyte globulin, which was less successful than the first. Several treatments were then tried and my spleen was removed *(E.K. had become refractory to platelet transfusions, and splenectomy was performed at a time when platelet counts were very low).*

In 1985, I suffered painful haemolytic attacks and was diagnosed with paroxysmal nocturnal haemoglobinuria, which lowered my haemoglobin values still more. Erythropoietin *(which had been developed in the meantime)* transiently helped, so that I did not need any transfusions. Cyclosporin A was also tried *(but had to be stopped because of kidney damage and severe hypertension. E.K., with a remarkable will-power, learned to live with a haemoglobin value around 5 g%, doing regular physical exercise, refusing transfusions).*

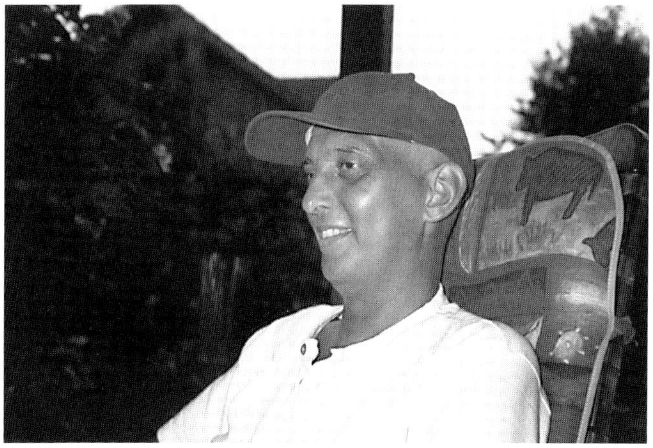

**Fig. 1.** Patient E.K., May 1999, 3 weeks after bone marrow transplantation from an unrelated donor.

During that period, I felt really well. In 1998, I was diagnosed with myelodysplastic syndrome, and *(since the percentage of blasts increased rapidly)* I was given bone marrow in May 1999 *(from an unrelated donor, after con-*

KARGER

Fax + 41 61 306 12 34
E-Mail karger@karger.ch
www.karger.com



0001–5792/00/1031–0063$17.50/0

Accessible online at:
www.karger.com/journals/aha

Catherine Nissen, MD
Department of Research, University Hospital
CH–4031 Basel (Switzerland)
Tel. +41 61 265 23 33, Fax +41 61 265 23 50
E-Mail nissen@magnet.ch

*ditioning with VP16, cyclophosphamide and TBI. After very severe complications during the early post-transplantation phase, he rapidly recovered and was discharged 3 weeks after transplantation).* Today, 4 months after transplantation, I feel completely healthy at the age of 44.

Without Prof. B. Speck, his team and my entire confidence, all this probably would not have happened. Prof. Speck took care of me and my disease for over 20 years, and I am greatly indebted to him.

## Comments

E.K. was lucky

- to be diagnosed with severe aplastic anaemia at a time when antilymphocyte globulin had just become available as a treatment alternative for patients who did not have a matched sibling donor for bone marrow transplantation, and
- to survive a long period of pancytopenia until erythropoietin and cyclosporin became available, and matching techniques for selection of unrelated donors were improved.

He was wise to refuse transfusions over all the years, since, being previously heavily transfused, engraftment of the unrelated bone marrow could have been compromised, and iron overload or acquisition of hepatitis C could have caused irreversible organ damage.

The success of the unrelated bone marrow transplantation after a 22-year history of therapeutic trial and error was hardly predictable. The case of E.K. illustrates how being 'off protocol' can be a chance by provoking experimental treatment. For E.K., the development of new therapeutic tools and strategies has kept pace with the natural history of his disease. Though few patients may be as lucky, it is encouraging to know that in severe aplastic anaemia, even in an apparently desperate situation, the outlook is never hopeless.

Acta Hæmatologica

Acta Haematol 2000;103:65

# Outlook

The beginning and the end of Bruno Speck's scientific career were milestones in the history of severe aplastic anaemia (SAA). In the early 70s, when Bruno Speck became involved with SAA, the disease had just begun to emerge as a distinct entity with an invariably fatal outcome in its severe form. Though diagnosis was possible, the available therapeutic tools failed to alter the course of the disease; spontaneous remissions were extremely rare. Bone marrow transplantation (BMT) brought new hope. Bruno Speck set out to change the poor outlook for patients with SAA and to explore the use of antilymphocyte globulin (ALG) for patients not eligible for BMT. Together with the haematology community, he achieved a major therapeutic breakthrough. Today, SAA has lost its stigma as a fatal disease, the prognosis for individual patients is excellent. However, many problems remain and we are again at a crossroads with the disease.

The near future may change our concepts of SAA, both in terms of the understanding of its pathophysiology and the development of new or more specific therapeutic tools. The solution to 'Damaschek's riddle', i.e. the cause for the close connection between SAA, paroxysmal nocturnal haemoglobinuria and myelodysplastic syndrome may become unravelled. New haematopoietic growth factors or new combinations of cytokines may turn out to be more effective than those currently in use. Prevention of apoptotic death of stem cells as a logical approach may prove beneficial. Stem cell transplantation as a curative treatment of SAA is developing rapidly. Traditional BMT has been supplemented by extension of the pool of potential donors and the detection of new possible sources of stem cells. Through rapidly expanding registries of unrelated donors and cord blood banks together with refined HLA typing and recognition of 'permissible' mismatches, it may soon become possible to find an appropriate stem cell graft for the majority of SAA patients. In addition, toxicity of the procedure is likely to be reduced by the use of low-intensity conditioning regimens in the near future, which may provide a 'graft-versus-aplasia' effect with less unwanted side-effects. The recent detection of cells in the brain capable of haematopoietic reconstitution opens a new experimental world: theoretically, the deficient haematopoietic stem cell pool in SAA might be restored by autochthonous stem cells, which are unlikely to be affected by the disease. Such an approach appears futuristic at the present time and may never be realized in the form that we now anticipate. However, looking at the fascinating history of ALG in retrospect, I conclude that the potential of 'new' possibilities is essentially unpredictable. Originally, ALG was thought to be beneficial in SAA by preventing rejection and graft-versus-host disease after transplantation of mismatched bone marrow. Only later did it become clear that ALG itself was the active principle as an immunosuppressant. Thus, the concept was wrong but the application right. The serendipity of investigators, collaboration of different teams involved in the investigation of the concept, the effort to collect international data, and creativity of the mind towards their correct interpretation contributed independently to the ultimate success of ALG. It is likely that future improvements in the treatment of SAA will depend on a similar 'mix of ingredients'.

*Alois Gratwohl*, Basel

KARGER

Fax + 41 61 306 12 34
E-Mail karger@karger.ch
www.karger.com



Accessible online at:
www.karger.com/journals/aha

Acta Hæmatologica

## Author Index Vol. 103, No. 1, 2000



## Subject Index Vol. 103, No. 1, 2000



KARGER
Fax + 41 61 306 12 34
E-Mail karger@karger.ch
www.karger.com



Accessible online at:
www.karger.com/journals/aha